STEREOSCOPIC ACUITY IN OCULAR PURSUIT OF MOVING OBJECTS

MATTHIAS & ULRICH SACHSENWEGER

Stereoscopic acuity in ocular pursuit of moving objects

Dynamic stereoscopy and movement parallax: relevance to road safety and occupational medicine

Reprinted from *Documenta Ophthalmologia*, Volume 78, Nos. 1–2 (1991)

Springer Science+Business Media, B.V.

Library of Congress Catalog Card Number: ac40-1560 (ISSN 0012-4486)

ISBN 978-0-7923-1486-8 ISBN 978-94-011-2572-7 (eBook)
DOI 10.1007/978-94-011-2572-7

MATTHIAS[1] & ULRICH[2] SACHSENWEGER
[1] *Schlehental 39, D-8300 Landshut, Germany*
[2] *Kühninchterweg 15, D-7700 Hoyerswerda, Germany*

Translation into the English language by W. Ghantus, Berlin.
Originally published by Akademie Verlag, Berlin as:
Das Raumshen bei bewegten Objekten auf der Basis der dynamischen Stereoskopie und der Bewegungsparallaktoskopie sowie seine Bedeutung für Arbeits- und Verkehrsmedizin, 1988, SAW, math.-nat.Kl-, Bd. 199, H:6. ISBN 3-05-500469-8

Contents

Preface

There has been growing acceptance of the insight that the methods so far used in the testing of visual functions have been inadequate when it comes to specific problems and should, therefore, be supplemented with more specialised methods for dynamic testing. As long as two decades ago, large-scale mass screening produced evidence to the effect that visual acuity, so far exclusively determined by means of still samples, was not identical with visual acuity in the ocular pursuit of moving targets (dynamic visual acuity). In other words, vision testing can, at present, provide little information on an individual's capability of identification, appreciation, and judgement of mobile objects.

Spatial, three-dimensional perception of moving targets, hereafter referred to as dynamic stereoacuity, is the particular subject on which findings are reported in this article. Findings of that kind are of considerable relevance to everyday life, since many of the phenomena that have to be three-dimensionally perceived in private life and in occupational practice, are in movement. So far, dynamic stereoacuity has never been systematically studied and is still a blank space on the maps of ophthalmology and physiology. This is equally true for dynamic stereoscopy in binocular vision as well as for perception on the basis of movement parallax, a phenomenon of differentiated contour displacement within a given field of vision which is also available to the monocular individual under conditions of head or body or object movement within the visual space.

Since 1984, growing attention has been paid to dynamic vision in the context of medicine for traffic safety to reduce the rate of road accidents as well as in the context of occupational health with partiular reference to ergophthalmology for certain occupational fitness categories, and also in connection with medicine in sport to optimise top sporting performance, to mention only a few examples. Hence, some interest can be expected, not only among ophthalmologists, for results recorded from studies into and analyses of dynamic three-dimensional perception, its potentials and normal values, and also for possible testing procedures, disorders, and inhibitory factors.

This article is intended to enlarge the knowledge about dynamic visual acuity compiled in previous publications and to offer clues for testing and evaluation to readers who are particularly interested in the two modes of dynamic stereoscopic vision. It may possibly prove helpful in providing encouragement for further investigations into dynamic performance of the visual organ.

Dr. sc. med. Matthias Sachsenweger was in charge of the design of the binocular rotational prismometer and investigations into dynamic stereoscopy. Design of the parallactoscopometer and studies into dynamic parallactoscopy were conducted by Dr. med. Ulrich Sachsenweger.

Rudolf Sachsenweger

1. Introduction

Three-dimensional perception of moving objects (dynamic stereoacuity) plays an important part in quite a few occupational and non-occupational every-day activities. It has, nevertheless, been ignored in ophthalmological practice and occupational health care, although, in recent years, testing of dynamic vision has been recommended by growing numbers of expert bodies on an international scale. Specialised studies into dynamic stereoscopy are still lacking altogether. All investigations so far undertaken into dynamic visual acuity have shown that conclusions cannot be readily drawn as to vision with moving targets from any of the testing procedures that have been used up to now.

There are two factors of stereoscopic vision that were found to relate to dynamic three-dimensional perception: dynamic stereoscopy on the basis of a transversally disparate image of the object in both eyes and dynamic parallactoscopy applicable to cases of monocularity. The latter results from the apparent displacement of contours in the course of motion. This paper has been written for the purpose of describing hardware for threshold determination of either visual power, as well as for expounding normal values and presenting optimum test conditions and, finally, elucidating the causes for the impairment of either variant of vision.

*

So far, there have been neither fundamental studies nor testing methods in the context of dynamic stereoacuity, i.e. stereopsis in the ocular pursuit of moving targets. This is quite a surprising shortcoming, since many things visually perceived by human beings are in three-dimensional movement in their general and specific occupational environment, and the correct assessment of such targets of vision is of crucial importance in many situations.

Three purposes have been defined for the visual organ in its association with the overall organism by F.B. Hofmann (1925), a sensory physiologist: guidance of the individual in controlled movements, orientation in space, and transmission of knowledge about exogenic phenomena and, thus, support of spiritual education. Visual perception of objects in the processes of movement is associated with each of these three purposes. Such orientation about details in space calls for a very high level of associative evaluation of optosensorial impressions. It also requires, of course, a general disposition to three-dimensional thinking which may be impaired, for example, in individuals with cerebral damage (Rennert, 1977).

The capability of the accurate location of moving objects has been formed in a stepwise manner through extended periods of phylogenesis. Three-dimensional visual perception of moving objects has been essential in numerous situations including the appraisal of prey and adversary, escape, avoidance of obstacles, hunting, etc. The performance of the visual organ was adjusted to the performance of locomotoricity, which, with modern technology, however, no longer applies to the complexity of life.

Vision and movement are closely related to each other in human everyday life, although they are tested separately for reasons of practicability in ophthalmological examinations – not really to the benefit of the reliability of findings – not to mention Hering's fall test (1879) in which movement is more or less constant and is associated with the velocity and acceleration of fall, an approach abandoned a long time ago because of its inadequacy.

Tests in which immobile optotypes are still used as targets are actually confined to static methods and are applied to something which is an extraordinary case of vision. This is true in many respects. Once such a test of visual acuity has proved to be sufficiently informative (Aulhorn, 1976); there have always been voices (Comberg, 1953; Schober, 1976) who have called for workplace-adjusted or traffic-related checks by ergophthalmological aspects and criteria, at least for special cases such as fitness assessment for special occupations. Dynamic visus testing was recommended by Methling and Wernicke (1969) with a view to analysing asthenopic complaints in the course of occupational activity.

It was not until 1984 that a WHO Working Group on the Role of Medical Factors in the Causation of Road Accidents asked for the enlargement and improvement of current testing procedures by adding dynamic vision testing in order to bridge the gap in our present knowledge (ICP/ADR 044.3551 E, 15 May 1984, WHO Regional Bureau for Europe). Extracts of the report read as follows: '(7.3) Conventional tests of static visual acuity . . . were not effective in predicting increased risk of accidents: however, it was realised that practical methods of testing for dynamic visual acuity and other aspects of vision which were important in this connection, had not yet been fully developed. (7.4) . . . It was recommended that the sponsoring of a study relating to this be considered.'

Aspects relating to dynamic vision in an occupational environment were discussed at an international ergophthalmological symposium held in Tampere, Finland, 1985, where preliminary steps were also taken towards testing for dynamic visual acuity in the context of top competitive sports. In 1985, testing for dynamic vision was demanded for some sport disciplines by a number of National Olympic Committees, including the US NOC.

The following three examples actually outline the three major applications of testing for dynamic vision in everyday life. They are medicine for traffic safety, occupational health with particular emphasis on ergophthalmology, and sports medicine. Dynamic vision is of importane at many more levels and to many more situations in everyday life. Sufficient evidence has been produced to the effect that there is by no means parallelism between the static and dynamic performances of the visual organ. This has been unambiguously borne out by all previous practices of testing for visual acuity in the ocular pursuit of moving targets (Jaeger and Honegger, 1964; Ludvigh, 1949; Ludvigh and Miller, 1958). Dynamic visual acuity may even be superior to static visual acuity when it comes to low-speed motions (Schober, Munker, and Grimm, 1967). The same may apply to certain forms of nystagmus and to visual field impairment (Jaeger and Honegger, 1964). Inter-individual variation of test results has been of considerable dimensions in that context, and has not been in conformity with the usual amount of variability in routine visual acuity checks in general ophthalmological practice (Honegger, 1966).

One particular role is played by two optosensorial components in dynamic three-dimensional perception, binocular stereoscopy, and kinetoparallactoscopy which is also effective in cases of monocularity. Stereoscopy is based on transversally disparate reflection in either retina of the object of fixation as well as on binocular fusion in the striated, parastriated, and peristriated areas. It is characterised by the high reliability of visual perception, as well as by remarkable accuracy, coming very close to the high precision of vernier visual acuity (Heinsius, 1964). Dynamic parallactoscopy, on the other hand, is also effective with monocularity. It is based on the apparent movement of contours within the field of vision along with an active or passive movement and is much coarser than stereoscopy. There are many possible situations in everyday life and occupational practice where dynamic parallactoscopy has little or no influence on three-dimensional perception. It is, however, clearly superior to stereoscopy for fast movements and long distances. When it comes to ocular pursuit of moving objects in real life, movement parallax is supported and accompanied by additional, empirical or secondary factors of three-dimensional perception, such as linear and air perspectives, size ratios, overlapping contours or colour, and brilliance phenomena.

Any kind of dynamic vision has not only to make use of the centres and association tracks for stereopsis but also of extensive oculomotoric control systems in the cerebrum and mesencephalon. Ocular pursuit of moving targets consequently depends on additional factors. This may be clearly seen from quite a few systematic studies into monocular dynamic visual acuity, the earliest of which was published by Ludvigh (1949) and by Ludvigh and Miller (1958). Studies in the German-language on the same subject were primarily conducted by Jaeger and Honegger at the Department of Ophthalmology at Heidelberg University between 1958 and 1970. Their findings regarding the quality of visual acuity in the course of absolute or relative movement, have provided a good basis for studies into dynamic stereoacuity.

The importance of dynamic monocular visual acuity and dynamic stereoacuity in road safey and occupational medicine has steadily grown in recent years and will probably continue to grow. A rapid increase in road traffic density, new occupational requirements, and growing speed at shop-floor level are some of the reasons why occupational failure may have an affect on people with inadequate stereopsis and, even more, on individuals with reduced dynamic stereopsis. The associated ergophthalmological aspects are quite obvious: higher accident rates, impairment of occupational performance, reduced working speed for individually perceived sensorial insecurity and objectively existing weakness of performance, accumulation of job-related mistakes, etc. High-quality dynamic stereoacuity is essential in some top competitive sports, including all ball games. There are numerous sports where top performance can be ruled out without top-level dynamic stereoacuity. Monocular competitors, for example, would have no chance at all.

Remarkably differentiated and even contradictory terms and definitions are used to describe three-dimensional vision in the German and English languages (Bishop, 1975). 'Stereoscopy', 'stereoscopic visus', and 'stereoscopic depth perception' are but three of them. Westheimer (1979) spoke of the 'spatial sense of the eye' and had in mind the resolution power of the optic organ. In recent times, the term 'stereoscopy' has been generally confined to vision on the basis of transverse disparation, i.e. to differentiated horizontal reflection of an object in the retinae of both eyes, consequently, on the basis of position parallax. The other terms have usually been associated with the category of empirical or secondary stereopsis (spatial vision; Blake, 1977). Consequently, stereoscopy may result exclusively from binocular vision rather than from monocularity. 'Depth acuity' is usually the term for describing the quality of stereoscopic vision, although 'stereoacuity' (stereoscopic acuity, binocular stereoacuity, stereo visual acuity) appears to be much more unambiguous.

'Dynamic parallactoscopic vision', too, has occasionally been semantically attached to the overall term of stereoscopy, although it has nothing to do with the latter, since it is not exclusively linked to binocular vision; rather, it is available to the monocular individual, as well. On the other hand, 'parallactoscopy' has often been equalled to 'stereoscopic vision', since stereoscopy, after all, is based on position parallax of both eyes. In other words, phenomena or objects which, in the context of movement parallax, are consecutively perceived from two different positions of one eye, are simultaneously perceived by both eyes.

The term 'movement', too, is somehow burdened with ambiguity. Jaeger (1958), with reference to earlier ambiguous definitions, called the subject of his studies 'visual acuity for moving objects'. 'Movement of a watched object', however, can be passive just as it can be active. For this very reason, Schober, Munker, and Grimm (1967) chose the term 'dynamic visual acuity' but added that 'kinetic visual acuity' was the formulation used by other authors (Gramberg-Danielsen, 1976).

An analysis of terms used in the literature supported the use in this article of the terms 'dynamic stereoacuity' to define depth acuity with regard to moving objects and 'kinetoparallactic stereoacuity' to define the quality of stereopsis on the basis of movement parallax.

The investigations described in the following sections were primarily undertaken for the following reasons:

- development and verification of methods suitable for quality testing of dynamic stereoacuity and kinetoparallactic stereoacuity;
- analysis of both functions and their variations through the application of new instruments and tests on normally sighted persons;
- determination of the optimum conditions for testing;
- examination of either function for the effects of impairment of optosensorial perception.

2. Elements of dynamic stereoscopic vision

2.1 Monocular dynamic visual acuity

Visual acuity is used in both passive and active movement, because the head and body of any individual are in a constant state of steady movement. Nevertheless, the movement factor has been ignored in the assessment of visual acuity in ophthalmological practice. Yet, the presentation of stationary optotypes has been accepted as an almost compelling simplification in ophthalmological examination, although it has been generally admitted that there are substantial and individually highly divergent discrepancies between static visual acuity and visual acuity for moving objects. There is not even the slightest parallelism between the two in normally sighted persons or in persons with pathologically affected eyes.

Surprisingly, for a long time sensorial physiologists paid little attention to visual acuity in ocular pursuit of moving objects. The first systematic study into dynamic visual acuity, according to Honegger (1966), was conducted by Ludvigh during the Second World War, using naval aviator cadets. His results were surprising although the problem had been tackled earlier by Langmuir (1938). Visual acuity for moving objects, no doubt, can provide an important clue for a proper judgement of the visual organ and the upper limits of its capacity. Those early investigations and further post-war studies were comprehensively reviewed by Miller and Ludvigh (1962).

Ludvigh and co-workers also worked on the aesthesiophysiological foundations of dynamic visual acuity. In their investigations, emphasis was placed on the question of why visual acuity began to decline as soon as a target began to move, although the human eye is generally known to be capable of extremely fast movements. Yet, difficulties are obviously attached to the permanent, precise reflection in the foveola of a moving optotype, even more so as the tracing movements of the eyes are not in precise correspondence to the movements of the object, especially when those movements are circular (Gerathewohl, 1954). Much obviously depends on whether a moving object is permanently reflected in the foveola or extramacularly on the retina, the latter being the case primarily in response to fast movement. Also, the peripheral contrast was found to decrease if moving objects are involved (Methling and Wernicke, 1969). Therefore, it is not surprising that the decline in visual acuity for moving objects may be reduced by an intensification of luminance.

The first systematic approach to this problem, primarily in connection with ophthalmological questions, was made in Germany by Jaeger (1958–1969) and Honegger (1964–1970) and numerous co-workers at the Department of Ophthalmology at Heidelberg University. They defined dynamic visual acuity as visual acuity for moving objects (Honegger, 1966, 1970; Honegger and Alexandridis, 1970; Honegger, Kamschulte and Klein, 1970; Honegger and Schäfer, 1964, 1968a, b, 1970; Honegger, Schäfer and Jaeger, 1969; Jaeger, 1958; Jaeger and Honegger, 1964). Hence, scientific treatment has been given to almost all ophthalmological problems relating to dynamic visual acuity, and previously published results have been substantively enlarged and enriched.

Visual acuity declines in two phases when optotypes are moving: a slight initial decline up to angular velocities of something between 20 °/sec and 25 °/sec is followed by a relatively steep drop in visual acuity in response to higher angular velocities (Fig. 1). A remarkably wide scatter of dynamic visual acuity values, much higher than the scatter of values for static visual acuity, was recorded by Ludvigh (1949), even from normally slighted naval aviator cadets. Mean values recorded from emmetropic individuals with a static visus of 1.0 were found to vary by a factor of above 2 in response to 80 °/sec, according to Ludvigh and Miller (1958).

Conspicuously different results were obtained from investigations in which static and dynamic visual acuity had been compared: Weissmann and Freeburne (1965) found that up to 120 °/sec, persons with higher static visual acuity, were, on average, also better in dynamic visual acuity, although these findings were recorded from only three emmetropic probands. This is in contrast to the reports by Burg (1966) and Hübler (1964) as well as by Schober, Munker and Grimm (1967). These results are likely to suggest that static visual acuity, measured by common methods, does not really provide useful clues from which to deduce dynamic visual acuity. Dynamic visual acuity was found to be clearly reduced, even with average pedestrian speed.

Dynamic visual acuity, with particular referene to low velocities between 1 and 10 °/sec, was investigated by Schober, Munker and Grimm (1967) as well as by Söllner (1961) and Dehler (1967). Schober and co-workers used an apparatus for optotype projection by means of a rotary mirror. Other parameters were a 1.25 m observation distance, 60° overseeable angular range, and 25 cd/m^2 surrounding luminance. For a more accurate comparison of results, the static visual acuity of three test persons was adjusted to $V = 1.0$. Dynamic visual acuity was considerably increased up to an angular velocity of 3 °/sec, due to the absence of local adaptation, which, surprisingly, varies between individuals. That increase was followed by an even more unambiguous decline. The value of static visual acuity was restored at angular velocities of between 3 and 12 °/sec.

The following conclusions may be drawn from these general considerations:

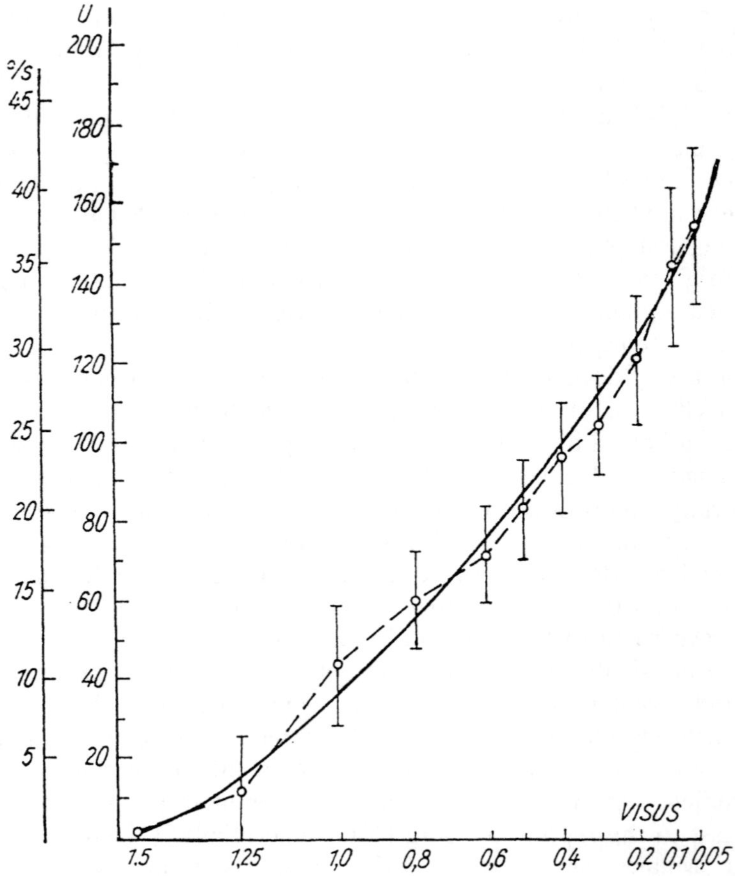

Fig. 1. Mean value curve of monocular dynamic visual acuity with scatter ($n = 10$). Abscissa: Decimal values of visual acuity. Ordinate: Revolutions per minute (rpm) and path in degrees per second.

1. Dynamic visual acuity is slightly above static visual acuity in response to low angular velocities around 3 °/sec.
2. Dynamic visual acuity clearly declines in response to higher angular velocities and accounts for no more than 50 to 10 percent of the static value, when 100 °/sec is reached.
3. It does not make much difference whether the optotype or the observer moves.
4. Even with angular velocity being used as a basis for comparison, the observation distance is believed not to be very important for the outcome of measurement.
5. Dynamic visual acuity in connection with binocularity is somewhat better than that relating to monocularity (Honegger, Schäfer and Jaeger, 1969).

6. Individuals of advanced age, on average are inferior to juvenile probands with regard to dynamic visual acuity, especially in the context of high velocities. On average, female probands are slighly inferior to male probands (Burg, 1964, 1965).

Hoogerhaide (1964) found a relative optimum to be paramacularly reached by dynamic visual acuity in the peripheral region of the retina in response to movements of 60 °/sec by virtue of the retinal structure. Peripheral visual acuity was studied by Low (1947) and Suzumara (1964) under conditions where optotypes were moved towards or away from the fovea: dynamic visual acuity was clearly better in the former case. Krot (1972) determined visual acuity using moving lines. According to Miller and Ludvigh (1962), vertically moved optotypes were more easily identified than horizontally moved targets. A theoretical analysis of movement and its effects upon visual acuity was made by Srinivasan and Bernard (1975).

2.1.1 Effects of mode of movement

A rotating prism of 4 pdpt, or an optotype projector, was used in most of the studies conducted by Jaeger and Honegger (1963/64). The prism is allowed to rotate in front of the projector at predetermined speeds accurately controlled by means of a tachometer. The image of a projected optotype is then deflected from the prism and is stimulated to circular movements. The threshold is determined by a gradual reduction, at any visual acuity stage, of the speed which is initially too high until the optotypes become identifiable, usually as Landolt circles. The system is then switched to smaller optotypes. Miller and Ludvigh (1962) converted revolutions to rate of motion per angular degree.

A horizontal display of moving optotypes is generally achieved by means of a rotating optotype projector and a semicircular projection screen (Honegger, Schäfer and Jaeger, 1969), even though, in most cases with a relatively short test distance. Eye movements have been recorded by means of oculography or a light beam reflected from the reflector of an eye contact lens and plotted onto photographic paper (Honegger and Schäfer, 1964). This has shown that horizontally moving optotypes are usually traced by sliding glances or small and jerky eye movements, with subtle variations in fixation being recorded from stoppage points. On the other hand, circular glances were found to be jerky with stoppage points and interruptions of movement, with the number of interruptions depending on speed. The slower the speed, the higher will be the frequency of the stoppage points.

Circular guidance movements, however, are never fully circular but have to have many leaps for correction. Eye muscles are possibly too coarsely coordinated for such movements. Circular eye movements tend to become increasingly inaccurate and to even deviate from the target, along with growing speed, and are eventually changed to real search movements. When it comes to velocities at which almost normal visual acuity is accomplished for the horizontal movement of optotypes (even larger optotypes will be identified much less easily) as soon as they are set to circular movement (Honegger, 1970).

A phase synchronism of glances with target movements is achieved at lower velocities, with the travel of the object image on the retina being limited, as soon as the radius of circular eye movements is reduced (Dieker and Honegger, 1968). However, at one and the same angular velocity, impairment of visual acuity in response to small circular movements is more drastic than in response to large movements, since the smaller circular movements are more difficult for the human eye to identify. Yet, surprising individual deviations from that rule may occur, especially in patients with pathological eye conditions.

The dynamic visual acuity generally achieved in response to horizontal movement was found to be four times higher than that for circular movement, if the path was taken as the point of departure (measured in degrees per second).

2.1.2 Dynamic visual acuity due to eye alterations

Almost all the knowledge so far accumulated on dynamic visual acuity in the case of eye alterations, has emanated from investigations conducted by Jaeger and Honegger (1964) and their coworkers.

The factor by which visual acuity is reduced has proved to be of crucial importance, particularly to myopers, when it comes to higher, uncorrected fields of refraction. Aphakial persons are no longer at a disadvantage to normally sighted individuals with the same static visual acuity when watching moving targets. Central scotomas of smaller dimensions are less of an obstacle to dynamic visual acuity which, anyway, depends more strongly on parafoveal retinal areas than static visual acuity. Relatively poor visual acuity values with rotating prisms have been recorded in cases of annular scotoma, since the perimacular regions of the retina are important to dynamic visual acuity for circular movements as well as to enlarged concentric visual field defects and hemianopsia with a vertical line of limitation.

The visual field may be experimentally narrowed for horizontal tracing movements up to 40 or even 50 degrees, without causing any decline in dynamic visual acuity (Honegger and Schäfer, 1970). This finding has proved to be of relevance in patients with visual field contraction who may apply for a driving licence, since the driver's field of view through a windscreen is generally limited by the front frame of the car (Schüler and Mürmel, 1979). The above studies have generally shown that only a small role is played by the visual field in the context of dynamic visual acuity, unless visual field contraction is accompanied by major abnormalities of a different nature.

Dynamic visual acuity was surprisingly found to be somewhat better than static visual acuity in individuals with congenital nystagmus. Nystagmus patients were even found to be noticeably superior to normally sighted persons when it came to high velocities. This may explain why nystagmus patients seem to be less handicapped in everyday life than they might be assumed to be on account of their static visual acuity.

Asynchronism of ocular muscles, for example, in patients with multiple sclerosis, cerebral commotio, and after alcohol intoxication, may substantively impair visual acuity for moving objects, even in the absence of ocular palsy (Honegger, 1970). Yet, the trend towards gradual normalisation is extraordinarily high.

Visual acuity for moving objects has proved to depend considerably on the adaptation of the eyes (Honegger and Alexandridis, 1970). Increase in angular velocity is inversely proportional to dynamic visual acuity (which declines). In other words, a decline in the latter will be less strongly pronounced when accompanied by growing adaptation luminance, provided that the simultaneously moving field of adaptation is large enough for the uninterrupted and homogeneous adaptation of the central retina. That supporting effect of adaptation luminance on dynamic visual acuity does not arise in a smaller field.

The quality of dynamic visual acuity in connection with eye raising and lowering may be of practical importance in certain cases. Aircraft pilots, for example, and, to a lesser extent, car drivers quite often have to gaze downwards or upwards and downwards to watch instrument panels. The common forward gaze in vehicles usually goes along with slightly lowered eyes. Visual acuity for moving objects was found to be at its best with a straight-ahead orientation of gaze (Honegger and Schäfer, 1968), with a more pronounced elevation or depression of gaze having an adverse impact upon visual acuity, since optosensory performance tends to be negatively affected by the need for a thorough coordination of movements of all six ocular muscles. In this context, elevation is more severely impaired than depression. A 5 degrees depression of gaze is considered to be the mean or optimum position of the eyes. In people of advanced age, a decline in visual acuity tends to be much more severe with vertical or oblique gaze directions. Coordination of horizontally acting extraocular muscles is obviously the least-complicated activity with a minimum effect upon sensomotory performance.

2.2 Stereoscopic vision

All stereoscopic perception is based on the lateral disparate imaging of an object within the field of vision in the retinae of both eyes. However, an additional role is played by movements for fixation and eye oscillations, mainly because stereoacuity is very much smaller than the diameter of a retinal cone. It is, therefore, absolutely essential to include the smallest micro-variations of fixation to find an explanation for the surprising precision of stereoacuity. Such subtlety can hardly be explained under static conditions (Adamson, 1951; Ditchburn and Ginsborg, 1953). Laterally disparate perception or reception is recorded in the cuneus of the visual cortex or striate area and is then communicated to other cerebral areas.

In physiology and ophthalmology, other attempts to explain stereoscopic vision have been more or less abandoned and, in many cases, are no longer mentioned, e.g., morphogenetic processes or psychic factors. Yet, the so-called central factor proposed by Hofmann (1924) has been fully accepted and, thus, so has the dependence of binocular vision on highly complicated systems of a central nervous association. These systems are hard to analyse, since they have developed to an enormous complexity in man, and animal experiments are difficult to carry out in these areas (Keidel, 1976). It is because of these central nervous associations that the time required for stereoscopy is 10 times longer than is needed for mere recognition. The quality of depth perception is likely to grow along with the intensity of competitive phenomena between the two eyes.

'Nasal or non-chiasmatic disparity' has been used to describe the perception of objects further away than the point of fixation, whereas 'temporal or chiasmatic disparity' has been used to define the reception of objects closer to the percipient than the point of fixation. Points or objects subjectively perceived to be equally distant from the eyes are imaged on what are called identical retinal loci. Good stereoscopic vision has proved to depend on the projection, in what is called Panum's fusional area, of objects imaged in lateral disparity. Stereoscopic vision is only slightly reduced or not reduced at all by fixation disparity (Crone, 1973).

Haploscopic vision, resulting experimentally or artificially from a fusion of two images with laterally disparate details, should be distinguished from the term 'stereoscopic vision in free space'. The presence of sensory fusion is not necessarily a condition for stereoscopic vision (Bourdy, 1974; R. Sachsenweger, 1958).

The view has been expressed by a majority of authors that the visual percepts of either eye are associated, in an alternating way in the visual cortex, to the generation of a stereoscopic percept (Aulhorn, 1971; Dowrick, 1975; Forde and MacKinnon, 1975; Tyler and Sutter, 1979; Ueberschaar, 1975). In this context, Herzau (1976) found the maximum interval to be somewhere between 400 and 500 milliseconds and the minimum interval to be 190 milliseconds.

Movements of gaze are not actually necessary to provide a stereoscopic percept (von Tschermak, 1931). However, they may be of some importance in strengthening the plasticity of a visual percept. A given object of vision is actually scanned by gaze movements. Yet, a general three-dimensional percept may be generated, even in flash lighting, during which eye movements are not really thinkable.

Stereoscopic vision has been gradually enhanced in quality in the course of phylogenesis. Stereoscopy, after all, is based on a partial cross-over of the optic nerve tracks in the chiasma, and animals without chiasmatic cross-over, such as birds, are not capable of genuine stereoscopic vision. The phylogenesis of mammals has been characterised by a gradual translocation of the eyes from the lateral to frontal position, with simultaneous retroplasia of the snout. Fields of vision have been gradually and more widely overlapping. This has enlarged the basis for stereoscopy. Highly advanced animals have additionally developed intra-retinal regional specialisation in the form of the fovea (optosensory centralisation) which has resulted in a higher accuracy of eye motility and, consequently, a more precise fixation (bifixation, according to Avetisov, 1978). Beasts of prey, for example, have excellent stereoscopic vision, thus reducing the potential advantages of mimicry and immobility provided to their prey. Phylogenesis of vision has been additionally characterised by a comprehensive reorganisation of the visual centres in the central nervous system.

The retinocerebral optic nerve fibres are capable of extremely accurate projections of binocular percepts into the visual cortex and actually end in identical cortical cells. In lower mammals, the major centres of vision are still localised in the mesencephalon. The nerve track across lateral geniculate colliculi to the visual cortex only came into being during the course of further development and was accompanied by a consecutive decline in the role played by mesencephalic centres of vision (Fox, 1977; Pettigrew, 1979). The surface of the visual cortex has undergone continuous broadening, a process associated in man with the perfection of eye-hand coordination and the development of upright carriage and walking. Binocular vision with frontally orientated visual axes was to assume substantial importance in this phase of evolution.

Bishop (1975), on the other hand, suggested that stereoscopy had been the only advantage phylogenetically provided to pay for the loss of wide-ranging panoramic vision. This is typical, for example, in the rabbit with its laterally directed axes of the eyes. Animals without stereoscopic vision get along with successive parallax (Frey, 1953), i.e. to-and-fro movements of head and body. Such permanent movements are quite obvious in many species, such as birds, snakes, and fish.

The timing of the maturity of stereoscopic vision in children was found to vary with the different methods used in testing. Normal performance has not usually been recordable before late into the first decade of age, if the method required the cooperation of the infantile proband. On the other hand, stereoscopic vision was positively recordable, if visual performance was analysed by means of visually evoked cortical potentials (VECP), from the visual cortex, suggesting that the development had obviously been completed after the third year of age (Andree, 1977; Banks, Aslin and Letson, 1975; Lyle and Bridgeman, 1959; Römhild, 1983).

Orientation in space is a specific way for determining a head-related coordinate system, as well as for defining object velocities, and for distinguishing between the optosensory perception of object movement and the perception of one's own movement. Such a preliminary analysis is undertaken by area 17 in the visual cortex, while area 18 is primarily involved in the perception of fast-moving targets and their localisation, although at a limited resolution power, with area 19 being responsible for the perception of slow-moving objects. Yet, here we are still faced with severe gaps in interpretation (von Seelen, 1983). Many issues have remained obscure in spite of micro-electrode recording which is available today. Yet, it has not been really helpful that a large number of micro-electrode recordings have been taken from individual visual cortex cells of rabbit, cat, and monkey (Bishop, 1975) and have produced results of limited applicability to man with his more advanced forms of binocularity.

Cell complexes with directional sensitivity in the striate area recorded from cat brain by David Hubel and Torsten Wiesel (1962) emitted much weaker impulses as soon as movements deviated from the lateral direction, i.e. from the horizontal parallax of both eyes. Fields of reception in the striate area are small, mutually overlapping areas receiving identical stimuli for both eyes, yet, with different intensities, for example, in the case of monocular dominance. They are capable of differentiating with astounding accuracy stimuli emitted from identical and laterally disparate retinal areas. The number of binocularly innervated neurons was found to drop along with amblyopia of one eye (von Noorden, 1979). Minor disparities in both eyes are accurately recorded by these fields. Westheimer and McKee (1979) concluded, from experiments using haploscopic line patterns, that stereoscopy was not based on the primary processing of monocular images but on the direct perception of disparity. Similar conclusions were drawn by Creutzfeld (1979). The stereooptic mechanisms are actually fore-connected to the centres of configurative or shape perception: An object has to be identified in three dimensions before its shape can be perceived (Baumgartner, 1978).

VECP diagnosis has become increasingly popular because of its noninvasive nature and has made major contributions to the analysis of central processes implied in binocular vision. Higher amplitudes with VECP were also recorded by Harter, Towle, Zakrewski and Moyer (1977) as well as by other authors from binocular and an equally strong stimulation of corresponding areas. A VECP amplitude with binocular observation was found to be somewhere between 25 and 30 percent of the total of monocular responses. Quite remarkably, that phenomenon was absent in cases of strabism. Laterally disparate stimulation within Panum's areas, too, led to an increase in amplitudes in the context of binocularity (Florentini and

Maffei, 1970; Regan and Spekreijse, 1970). That rise in amplitude was not recorded in stereoblind individuals. The relative density of cortical binocular stereoprojection in the immediate vicinity of the fovea was investigated by Friedburg (1980), using VECP with random dot stereotests and growing lateral disparity. He found the accuracy of stereoscopic discernibility to decrease with increasing lateral disparity.

The results obtained from VECP, on account of the structure of random dot patterns and point size, apart from anything else, have proved to be much too general for the proper measurement of stereoacuity. Against the background of the latest technological developments, the resolution threshold of VECP in response to stimulation with patterns of variable lateral disparity, was found to be about 2.5 arc minutes (Teping and Pesch, 1984). However, something between 5 and 40 arc seconds can be reached by a normally sighted individual with normal stereoacuity.

There is a well known dominance of the left cerebral hemisphere for speech-related information and associated functions. The right cerebral hemisphere, on the other hand, prevails in processing binocular visual information and has, consequently, connected to it the functions of three-dimensionality (Levy and Lawson, 1978). In practice, however, there are many deviations from that principle of laterality (Lehmann and Julesz, 1978). For example, fusion, on the one hand, and stereoscopy, on the other, are controlled by different neuronal mechanisms. That is why fusion capacity is not a conclusive indicator of the quality of stereoacuity (de Decker and Scheffel, 1978).

2.2.1 *Determination of static stereoacuity*

Elementary knowledge about stereoscopic vision and stereoacuity may be traced back to the Middle Ages. In modern physiology and ophthalmology, interest in stereoacuity has been of surprisingly recent origin, although all the conditions existed for its analysis and testing.

In Central Europe, prior to the turn of this century, the so-called triple-bar test was used by the physiologists Hering and von Helmholtz to demonstrate stereoacuity (depth acuity). It had also been accepted as a standard procedure in ophthalmology, and has retained this position ever since, although more modern techniques, including polarisation and anaglyphic plotting, have been introduced in ophthalmology and occupational medicine, mainly over the last decade. Yet, as far as precision is concerned, these approaches are not even remotely competitive to the triple-bar system. Hering and von Helmholtz never published anything about the triple-bar apparatus which was first publicised by Hummelsheim in 1905. Pfalz (1907) introduced it to a wider public. The rig was made up of three steel pins of different thicknesses which were vertically placed and could be moved in front of, or behind, their common frontal plane. The person being tested was required to adjust the three pins or bars into one frontal parallel and to comment on their relative depth arrangement.

This method has been modified many times in recent years. The most important modifications were made by Cords (1912), Davidson (1935), Kessler (1947), Langlands (1929), Litinsky (1936), Perlia (1911), Pfalz (1907), Verhoeff (1933) and Woodburne (1934). Two, instead of three bars were used by Howard (1919) and Matsubayashi (1937). Mehlhose (1975) tried to improve the handiness of the apparatus in ophthalmological practice by means of an electrical remote control. The apparatus designed by Römhild (1983) contained three blackened wires (0.3 mm in diameter = 2′17″ in aperture angle) for a test distance of 45 cm. The two outer wires could be moved horizontally, relative to their common plane, by means of a micrometer screw.

The natural conditions for vision, using real objects of vision, and the impossibility of any guesswork, say, due to proportional sizes, linear perspective, and convergence, are considered to be the most important advantages of the triple-bar system (Haase, 1980).

Another testing method by which to measure stereoacuity, called the fall test, was mentioned by Hering as early as in 1879. He dropped a ball in front of or behind a vertically suspended thread, and the proband was asked to comment on the localisation of the ball. The system was still given a high rating by Bielschowski in 1923. It has now been entirely abandoned as having too many shortcomings, and it is only mentioned here because a ball is an object moved by velocity of fall which requires three-dimensional assessment.

A remarkable role for the measurement of stereoacuity was played by haploscopic procedures, above all, lens stereoscopes, in the first half of the 20th century. Pulfrich's stereoscopic silhouette chart is a good example (1911). Yet, since the visual conditions at a stereoscope are of an artificial nature, some test on probands with normal stereoscopic vision tend to partially or totally fail. Similar assessments have been valid for other haploscopic instruments. Also, there have been very few correlations between the test results obtained with real targets, on the one hand, and those recorded from haploscopic procedures, on the other (Chevaleraud, Brenneisen and Santucci 1975; Holland, 1960; Römhild, 1983), since demands in terms of sensory physiology differed too greatly.

The measurement of static stereoacuity was greatly updated prior to and during the Second World War, for example, when the split-bar instrument was invented by Best (1949) and the stereo-eidometer by Monjé (1949).

With modern, post-war methods, a stereoscopic percept is generated by using polarisation or anaglyphic haploscopy to assign to each of the two eyes one detail of an image in lateral disparity. Methods of this kind are sufficient for ophthalmological practice and even provide major benefits, such as easily intelligible test problems, fast testing, and easier handling of the test in book form. Yet, some setbacks have been implied. For example, they do not enable testing of stereoacuity up to the limits of stereoscopic capability. The stereoscopic percept is artificially generated, and certain probands may have problems in their perception of a simulated three-dimensional situation. So-called stereo-retardation has quite often occurred, i.e. considerable individual discrepancies regarding the time which passes before the image details perceived in lateral disparity merge into one stereoscopic percept. Such retardation may last up to 15 seconds, but is unknown when probands are exposed to natural three-dimensional situations. A great diversity of stereoscopic optotypes is used in modern testing. Many of them do not even meet the elementary demands of optical density and contrast.

Random dot patterns are being used on a steadily increasing scale (Aschenbrenner, 1954; Julesz, 1964; Shipley, 1971). However, the results obtainable from these tests were found to be highly heterogeneous (Campos and Enoch, 1980; van Lear, Blum and Niesel, 1982; Reinecke and Simon, 1974; Westheimer and McKee, 1979). The stereoscopic threshold in the context of random dot tests is obviously higher than that associated with real optotypes, because dots rather than contours are involved. Dot size and dot configuration are essential to identification. Real depth differences are used in the Frisby test (Frisby, Mein, Saye and Stanworth, 1975) which is primarily applied to children examined for orthoptic judgement. Doege and Krause (1977) tried to introduce a raster or grid separation procedure to test binocular functions. Stripe grids could be substituted by cylindrical lens grids. Random dot test grids were also found to be applicable (Lang, 1983).

With more recent test procedures, emphasis is laid on practicability. Both ophthalmologists and works medical officers and other specialists in occupational medicine need good results from practicable stereoscopic testing methods and from which the existence or approximate quality of stereoacuity can be established. Hence, in this context, determination of individual upper limits of stereoscopic performance would be less important than immediate information on the presence or absence of stereopsis.

Obviously, there have never been any attempts to test stereoacuity in ocular pursuit of moving objects. All methods and equipment so far known have been used for testing at rest, except for Hering's fall test (1879).

2.2.2 *Quality of stereoacuity*

Stereoacuity (depth acuity) was measured for the first time by v. Helmholtz who discovered that the threshold of lateral disparity was 60″. He erroneously concluded that normal visual acuity and stereoacuity should be more or less identical. Nevertheless, he was not entirely wrong, if one considers that one angular minute has long ceased to be recognised as a normal value of visual acuity.

Lower threshold values have recently been found by many authors.

Lateral disparity angles between 1.89 and 5 angular minutes were recorded by Howard (1919) from 25 persons tested, while Teichner, Kobrick and Wehrkamp (1955) recorded values of 0.47 and 0.11″. Values below 2″ were also found by Anderson and Weymouth (1923) as well as by Langlands (1929). Optimum stereoacuity ws rated to be 2″ by Scott and Masch (1974).

Closer consideration of measurements taken of special categories of occupational activity, are likely to suggest that a threshold from 5 to 10″ should be rated as very good, while values between 10 and 30″ should be interpreted as normal or sufficient (Gehrke, 1965). Threshold values lower than 45″ can no longer be considered as normal. For triple-bar testing at a distance of 5 m to give a stereopsis of 20 mm, Frejman (1940) proposed the rating 1 (= normal or 10.5″). All other values might then be expressed in decimal fractions. It should always be borne in mind that stereoacuity values may strongly depend on apparatus and method. A stereoacuity of at least 8″ has been considered absolutely essential by Feldes and Römhild (1981) when it comes to the evaluation of stereoscopic aerial photographs for geodetic surveying and cartography. Litinski (1936) insisted on 10″ for pilot trainees, and Colajanni (1939) suggested 7.5″ for the same purpose. The lowered average stereoacuity of women in certain statistical records, might be attributable to lower average pupillary distance.

The real difference in assessment between depth-distant contours would naturally depend on the distance of a given optotype or visual object. In this context, real discernible depth distance tends to grow along with the square of distance. When depth distance was modified, most authors found identical or similar values for individual lateral disparity (Jameson and Hurvich, 1959; Micko, 1955/56; Ogle, 1958; Vesper, 1965). Yet, test conditions for comparative measurements in various distances should be kept constant, especially bar thickness, visual acuity for close and distant ranges, luminance of the residual field, and throughout the space of testing, etc. After all, there are individuals with striking discrepancies between near-field and far-field stereoacuity values (Römhild, 1983; M. Sachsenweger, 1984).

A range of up to 650 m may be covered by long-distance stereoscopic perception, according to Ueberschaar (1976), though in every-day practice, stereoscopic perception is considered to be of importance only up to 50 m, or only 20 m according to Hartmann and Stöcker (1983) or not more than 10 m according to Baumgartner (1978) and Gipson (1966). When it comes to longer distances, its importance is likely to decline in relation to the empirical factors of three-dimensional perception which are also at the disposal of monocular individuals.

If stereoacuity is checked by means of a triple-bar apparatus, the threshold adjustment of the central bar behind the common plane of all three will have to be smaller than in front of that plane for test distances of 4 to 5 m. The ratio will have to be the other way round for near-test distances, say, 30–40 cm. This, according to Hering-Hillebrand, is attributable to horopter circle deviation. The horopter circle is the frontal plane subjectively perceived by an observer and is concave, relative to the observer, for close-up fixation but convex for distant viewing. These are differences which add to the difficulties in a proper appraisal of test results. It is because of those difficulties that only one focus ahead has been chosen in most cases of modern stereoscoptic testing.

2.3 Dynamic parallactoscopy

Stereoscopic vision on the basis of movement parallax can be defined as the inevitable three-dimensional percept received by a monocular observer who is in movement relative to a number of visual objects within his or her own field of vision, for example, by head or body movements (active dynamic parallactoscopy) or by looking at moving objects (passive dynamic parallactoscopy). The latter may be experienced or simulated by animated movies (von Tschermak, 1947). The observer in such a situation will visually perceive the displacement of object contours relative to each other. Nearer objects will then move rapidly and in a counterdirection relative to the observer, while more distant objects, behind the point of fixation, seem to move slowly and almost in the same direction as the observer does. Objects at the same distance from the observer as the point of fixation appear to be immobile. The same effect will be generated if the observer moves forward (closer to the object): nearer targets apparently move towards the obsever at a growing speed or swerve to the right or left, while more distant targets appear to move in the same direction as the observer. The fixed target is thus not only perceived under optimum conditions of vision, i.e. most accurately, but also all additional objects can be easily differentiated from the object of fixation (Körner and Dichgans, 1968).

The three-dimensional percept on the basis of movement parallax is one of the empirical factors of stereoscopic perception and, consequently, is the result of a learning process. This is missing in small children. Kinetoparallactoscopic depth localisation, however, is involuntarily performed almost like a reflex. It is extremely difficult to measure its quality by accurate data, because it depends on several factors. An excessive three-dimensional percept may be generated, through movement parallax, by very fast movements and by watching movies. The kinetoparallactoscopic displacements of objects relative to each other within a given field of vision, are pseudomovements. Their identification requires a certain minimum speed, approximately corresponding to the limit value for the identification of different positions. Yet, there is also an upper speed limit, and if this is surpassed, identification of apparent positional variation will be hardly possible or will no longer be possible at all. In this context, a role is played by the distance between observer and object formation. Movements may be horizontal, vertical, or diagonal; displacements among objects in different distances from an observer will be identical with any kind of straight movement.

Dynamic parallactoscopy occurs along with active and passive movements, with the effect being one and the same in either case. Active movement defines any kind of movement of the observer's head or body, e.g., when walking or riding on horseback, likely to result in horizontal as well as vertical rhythmic, parallactic object shifting. Passive movement is caused by movement in a vehicle, its direction usually being horizontal. It may be vertical, as well, for example, when the observer is moving in an open elevator. A highly instructive example has been mentioned by von Tschermak (1938): A bar system, say, the collector arm of a streetcar, cannot be three-dimensionally perceived by an observer at a medium distance from the object by means of stereoscopy alone. However, a three-dimensional percept will be immediately created for a moving observer or as soon as the streetcar is started.

A three-dimensional percept on the basis of movement parallax, just as one in connection with stereoscopy, is created involuntarily and inevitably. Yet, theoretically, depth localisation is absolutely possible on the basis of thinking or an analysis of observation and with due consideration to velocity and apparent or factual direction of movement, say, by association of perceptions of concomitant = more remotely localised or lagging behind = more closely positioned.

In stereoscopy, on the other hand, the depth percept is based on position parallax of both eyes. Stereoscopy provides a three-dimensional percept of high accuracy, particularly of immobile objects, with the accuracy being about four times higher, compared to a three-dimensional percept obtainable from dynamic parallactoscopy. Intact binocular vision is a prerequisite for such stereoscopic vision. It is totally eliminated for long-distance vision (more than 650 m) and tends to fail when it comes to visual objects with horizontal contours if lateral disparate images are absent because of the horizontal position parallax of the two eyes. If, however, both means of judgement are available, i.e. stereoscopy and dynamic parallactoscopy, the latter will substantially support the former. According to von Tschermak (1938), three-dimensional vision may be enhanced by stereoscopy by at least 25 percent.

While three-dimensional vision on the basis of movement parallax has long been a well-known phenomenon, related terminology has continued to be remarkably heterogeneous. Von Tschermak (1938) spoke of 'parallactoscopy'. This term, however, is inaccurate, since stereoscopic vision, too, is based on a parallax – the so-called position parallax of both eyes which is in keeping with the pupillar spacing. The term 'time parallax' is used in astronomy to measure the distance of stars. Hence, the term 'parallactoscopy' does not cover the essential factor, movement. The term 'dynamic parallactoscopy' would be somehow more acurate for distinguishing position parallax from time parallax. The inaccurate definition of the term 'parallactic displacement' was deplored by Guist (1922) who conducted fundamental studies into the geometric background of such a displacement. The term 'kinetoscopic parallactoscopy' may be occasionally found in earlier publications.

The so-called depth acuity has nothing at all to do with the quality of stereoscopic vision, but is rather a term coined in photography and cinematography and is exclusively related to the imaging quality of a picture through a system of optical lenses, with due consideration of those three-dimensional distances in which the image is still sharply defined.

'Kinetoparallactic stereopsis' or 'dynamic parallactoscopy' appear to be the most suitable terms to describe three-dimensional vision on the basis of movement parallax.

There are many situations in which dynamic stereoscopy may compete with dynamic parallactoscopy and may perform much better than kinetoparallactic vision in the detection and identification of visual objects in a three-dimensional array near to the observer (Hartmann and Stöcker, 1983).

The most importance differences between dynamic parallactoscopy and dynamic stereoscopy may be seen from Table 1.

Table 1. Definitions of stereoscopy and dynamic parallactoscopy.

Form of stereoscopic vision	Stereoscopy	Dynamic parallactoscopy (kinetoparallactic stereopsis)
Threshold of visual performance	Steroacuity, Depth acuity	Kinetoparallactic stereoacuity
Mode of vision	Binocular depth localisation at rest and in movement	Depth localistion also monocularly possible; need for movement versus visual object
Contours	Dependent on vertical contours	Vertical, horizontal, and diagonal contours, depending on direction of movement (horizontal and vertical parallaxes)
Performance capacity	Static stereoacuity about 5–45″ lateral disparity, eliminated as of 650 m	Dependent on angle of viewing and relative depth difference; unlimited distance
Visual basis	Position parallax = pupillar spacing (simultaneous parallax)	Movement parallax, angle of viewing between initial and final position of movement (successive parallax)

2.3.1 Testing equipment

Surprisingly few instruments have so far been developed for qualitative determination of stereopsis on the basis of movement parallax, and they usually exhibit severe shortcomings. This differs drastically from the wide range of apparatus and methods available for the measurement of stereoacuity (depth acuity). Nearly all of them were developed in the first half of this century to define the degree of occupational incapacity (physical damage) due to a loss of one eye, and to determine possible compensation of binocular vision by movement of the head. This was required for expert medical opinion. Once that early period was over, few authors have dealt with dynamic parallactoscopy. This is the reason why all the devices and methods so far mentioned are neither suitable nor intended for testing of kinetoparallactoscopic performance under most varied aspects. All instruments so far available actually restrict possible movement to the extent of head movement, some of it being equivalent to a movement parallax up to 10 cm. This restriction actually rules out the quality assessment required for judgement of road traffic situations or occupational and sporting activities. These earlier methods are not even applicable to the scientific analysis of visual sensory performance of dynamic parallactoscopy.

An apparatus which could be used exclusively for expert assessment of monocular depth perception was described by Pfalz (1907). The worth of his stereo-optometer was disputed from the very beginning, primarily because tactile and positional perceptions played a role similar to the apparatus reported by Perlia (1911).

Cords (1913/14) described an experimental arrangement with which stereopsis could be qualitatively determined on the basis of parallactic displacement. His device was made up of two equilateral triangles, with their vertices being directed at each other (Fig. 3f). The lower triangle could be moved forward and backward. By looking through a slit, the proband had to assess the position of the two triangles. The viewing slit could be broadened for the additional determination of the movement parallax or for monocular vision, for which the head had to be moved to and fro. Horizontal head movements were recorded by a head-fixed printing device. The disadvantage of this arrangement was the use of diagonal contours which were hard to define and were individually different for their steroscopic valence.

Using this arrangement, Cords found that only a minor role was played by monocular depth perception with head movements up to 3 cm, whereas stereopsis was unambiguously improved by head movements of more than 3 cm.

For his studies into monocular dynamic parallactoscopy, Colenbrander (1949) used a triple-bar arrangement with a peri-ocular viewing slit which was different in width – up to 6 cm. To-and-fro head movements were permitted at any speed. The results of such tests depended on both side-to-side distance of the slit and monocular visual acuity. Under such experimental conditions, average binocular depth acuity was four times better than the threshold of monocular stereopsis supported by parallactic displacements through head movement. Film was also used by Colenbrander in his investigations of dynamic parallactoscopy by lateral moves of the film camera.

A parallactoscope, reported by sensory physiologist von Tschermak in 1938, was designed for ruling out all other factors of stereoscopic judgement and concentrating solely on the performance of dynamic parallactoscopy. It was particularly intended to rule out any three-dimensional percept on the basis of a static initial position without movement. With the parallactoscope, stereoscopic perception could only be accomplished by to-and-fro movement of the head. The design of that parallactoscope was preceded by an elementary apparatus which von Tschermak obviously used in his early studies into movement parallax. The apparatus was constructed from a square cardboard tube of about 10 cm, so that a proband could use both eyes. The tube had wires of different thicknesses inserted into it which were parallel to each other at different distances.

The parallactoscope, however, was good enough for more subtle examinations. It contained three vertically or horizontally adjustable parallel wire groups of four wires, each with viewing distances from 21 to 40 cm. The two outer wire groups were stationary. The central group was to be moved by the proband to appear in one frontal plane with the outer wires. The wires within the groups of four were spaced 5 mm apart, and the distance between groups was 14 mm. The background was alternatively black or white. The wire arrangement was illuminated from the side. The test configuration could be easily turned by 90 degrees to enable testing with the wires in a horizontal array. The viewing inlet was 12 cm in width and height. Head movement could be limited as necessary by means of lateral shields. Wires of different thicknesses and colour or different wire spacings could be chosen to avoid any impact of empirical factors of stereoscopic perception, especially a variation in size due to a closer approach.

This apparatus, too, was primarily intended for the measurement of the depth localisation capability of monocular probands with rhythmic head movement. The scatter of readjustments of head movements by monocular probands was found to be almost twice as much as that required by binocular individuals, although only for vertically set wires and horizontal head movements. Only minor differences were found to exist between monocularity and binocularity with horizontal wires and vertical head movements. Monocular stereopsis with no head movement was about 200 times poorer than that with a moving head. Without head movement, binocular adjustments were at least 25 percent better than the monocular value with horizontal head movements. Interpretation of the test results by von Tschermak (1938) was quite general and failed to enable a comparison to be made. His apparatus was obviously not used for mass screening. No information is available on the number of test persons or on the statistical calculations.

When probands were asked to move the central wires into one frontal plane with the outer wires, the central wires moved too far back in almost all cases. This is the common rule for stereoscopic vision due to the curvature of the horopter (see Section 2.2.2). That was difficult to explain for monocular vision, and von Tschermak failed to deal with this phenomenon in any great detail.

At medium velocities, three-dimensional perception on the basis of movement parallax was found to account for only one quarter of static stereoacuity (Colenbrander, 1949; Oloff and Podesta, 1937). Howard (1919) suggested the binocular threshold of depth perception by means of stereoscopy to be up to 20 times higher in accuracy than the monocular threshold on the basis of dynamic parallactoscopy. He mentioned a test instrument, the Howard-Dollman apparatus, with which, however, binocular vision was found to be three to four times better than monocular vision (Pierce and Benton (1975). According to Frey (1977), dynamic parallactoscopy is approximately comparable to an average output of stereoscopy, i.e. lateral disparity of 20 to 30″.

2.4 More empirical factors of stereoscopic vision

Apart from movement parallax, there are additional empirical (non-stereoscopic), so-called secondary factors of three-dimensional perception, such as perspective, visual size comparison, shadow casting variation of brightness and colour, or cover of objects. These factors are not tied to binocular vision and may be very accurate in certain cases. They are of great importance in everyday life.

The lateral disparate stereoscopic vision of man is predominant for distances of up to some 20 m. Empirical factors were shown to be of overriding importance to stereoscopic perception, even in individuals with binocularity, when it came to distances beyond 40 m. Either mode of vision may be equally valid, depending on the situation, between 20 and 40 m (Hartmann and Stöcker, 1983).

Empirical factors of depth perception have a considerable advantage in that they do not depend on intact binocularity and, consequently, can also become effective under conditions of monocularity. They may prove helpful to monocular individuals in finding their bearings in three-dimensional situations of everyday life. They relate to both moving and still objects, except for dynamic parallactoscopy (see Section 2.3) and, in special cases, they have proved to be highly instrumental in high-accuracy space judgement (Bishop, 1975).

It is by virtue of the geometric perspective (linear perspective) that all equidirectional lines within a given field of vision or in an image, tend to converge at one point, called the vanishing point. Apparent size and distance of the visual object are closely related to this phenomenon. Once the absolute size of a given object is known, the distance of its location can be approximately determined via the dimensions of its retinal image. The apparent distance of objects of unknown original size, viewed through a smaller visual angle, will be larger than that of the same objects when viewed through a wider visual angle. The three-dimensional percept is absolutely compelling, when objects of equal size but at different distances are compared to each other without any additional cues: The nearer object will appear to be larger to the observer.

The phenomenon of linear perspective means that a more distant object does not simply appear to be smaller to the percipient but is related to other object sizes. This is attributable to the fact that various retinal elements have only a relative rather than a fixed or absolute direction of vision assigned to them. They possess a capability of ordering or grouping rather than a high-stability value of measure or distance (von Tschermak, 1947). The overall sense of measure is shown to be crucially determined, not by objective distance, but by the imagination of the distance evoked in the percipient by the fixed object.

Aerial perspective is defined as a phenomenon, according to which, clouding tends to occur in the field of vision due to a growing thickness of air layers, depending on the levels of steam and dust, so that the sharpness of the contours tends to decline along with the growing distance of the object. The outlines of those objects, specifically their surface structures, will thus appear to be less clear to the observer, with coloration being changed to a blueish shade. It is a consequence of such a reduced marginal contrast that the outlines of nearer objects stand out darker against adjacent but more remote surfaces. Aerial perspective actually plays a great role in the three-dimensionality of the distant vision of objects in arrays.

The distribution of light and shadow, in conjunction with perspective, is a major cue for uniocular depth localisation. A pseudo-relief may quite frequently result from competition between light and shadow distribution or perspective, on the one hand, and lateral disparity, on the other. Light and shadow distribution has been used by many painters and graphic artists to create impressions of immense depth in their paintings. Brightness differentiation is also important in everyday life for identifying the bodily nature of an object: If, for example, a white surface is merely tilted by 0.5 degrees, the result will be a clearly discernible difference in luminance, and the surface will no longer appear plane.

A mutual overlapping of objects or intersection of contours, as far as they are clearly discernible, may provide unambiguous cues for positions of objects in space. They may prevent depth perception by stereoscopy and may well act as the most compelling factor in generating a three-dimensional percept in terms of 'nearer' or 'more distant'.

Distance perception is extremely poor on the basis of convergence and accommodation. Convergence cannot play a role until an object comes as close as 4 m (Hartmann and Stöcker, 1983). Even the fusing of very near objects with a clearly associated palpable stretching of the extraocular muscles can be helpful in generally estimating object distance at a very close range. Accommodation – in its own right – has been found to be completely unsuitable for estimating distances.

2.5 Dynamic vision

Slow movements of an object tend to evoke synchronous movements of ocular pursuit in the percipient, whereas high velocities are accompanied by saccadic eye movements with many corrective leaps. The threshold for perception of movement in the peripheral part of the retina was found to be lower than in the retinal centre, whereas the threshold for noticeability or peculiarity is higher in the periphery than in the centre. Almost all neurophysiological findings with regard to dynamic vision have so far been obtained by micro-recording from animals and can only be loosely applied to man who is characterised by more advanced ways of optosensory perception. The various types of apparent movements are associated with both retinal factors and those relating to the central nervous system.

An enormous amount of knowledge about the perception of movement has been accumulated over the past hundred years. A distinction is generally made between viewing real objects in movement with a travelling retinal image and stationary fixation and viewing immobile targets by a moving observer with ocular pursuit and, finally, combinations of both. Experimentally generated movement perception, too, may be of some relevance in studies into dynamic vision, for example, looking through a rotating prism, with simulated object movement, and apparent movements or after-images of movement.

Slow object movements cause movements of ocular pursuit which are synchronous with the speed of the visual object. Objects moving at faster speeds, say, up to 800 °/sec, evoke saccadic eye movements made by the percipient in an attempt to pursue the moving target. Different labels have been assigned to movements of ocular pursuit, including controlled movement, guided or accompanying movement, fixation of movement, pursuit movement at zero speed, or optically evoked and rhythmically controlled reflex.

The threshold for perception of movement, again, was found to be lower in the peripheral part of the retina than in the retinal centre, whereas the contrary applies to the threshold for noticeability or peculiarity. According to Schober, Munker and Grimm (1967), vision at very low speeds is somewhat better than visual acuity at rest (static visual acuity) and comes quite close to vernier acuity, which is thought to be attributable to the absence of local adaptation.

In the animal kingdom, dynamic vision, providing useful information on prey and enemies, is absolutely essential for the survival of any visually oriented creature. Phylogenetic development of dynamic vision, on account of its vital importance, has preceded phylogenesis in capability of pattern recognition. Recognition follows adjustment of fixation which may involve the entire body musculature. In man, this capability has been developed to different intensities and is believed to be very prominent in athletes (Miwa, Terado, Morita, Yamada and Zuzumura, 1972).

The theory of efference copy with intracerebral feedback processes and extraretinal signals, has often been used to explain the process of ocular pursuit movement in watching a moving object. On the other hand, MacKay (1970) and Noda (1975) found that a movement was perceived by the centres of visual perception only through a comparison of an object prior to and after eye movement.

Most of the neurophysiological knowledge about dynamic vision has been obtained from animal experiments and, thus, cannot be readily translated or applied to man (von Noorden, 1979), since major structures of visual pathways have undergone a change in the course of mammalian phylogenesis. Most of that change is characterised by gradual corticalisation. The majority of neurons in the visual cortex respond exclusively to moving stimuli. A generally accepted answer has obviously not yet been found to the question of the mode in man by which all neurons respond to various optical stimuli in different regions of the visual pathway (Sayk, 1979).

Optokinetic nystagmus was found to be closely associated with the perception of moving objects. Its morphology is unambiguous: a moving object is reflex-fixed in an attempt to achieve its constant reflection in the retinal foveola. Any retinal image movement leads to an assessment of the required gaze movement, which will eventually result in an ocular pursuit movement as a slow phase of optokinetic nystagmus, also referred to as the perception phase. The latter is presumably controlled via a subordinate sensomotor control circuit independent of human will. The eye snaps back to its initial position as soon as the end of the test path is reached (rapid phase of optokinetic nystagmus). As most of this process is of an involuntary nature, it becomes possible to objectively determine visual acuity. The existence of an involuntary urge of fixation as a result of automatic visuomotor control is important in the investigation of dynamic vision.

For any testing of movements, due attention should be given to the phenomena of apparent movements which may be based on both retinal and central visuosensory factors, with the impression of object movement being subjectively perceived only by the individual percipient. Apparent movements are predominantly associated with psychological parameters (Anstis, 1976). There is no doubt that this can lead to optical illusions of relevance to road traffic. Extended duration and stereotypy are the most important prerequisites for apparent movements.

There are two groups of apparent movements. One tends to give the impression that the point of fixation slightly approaches the observer (autokinetic effect). Apparent movements of that kind may also result, in certain cases, from a near-to-far or far-to-near shifting of the point of fixation. Apparent movements are also possible in the context of double image perception along with fusion or defusion attempts in the form of lateral moves towards or away from each other.

Dynamic after-images constitute the second group of apparent movements (Lehmkuhle and Fox, 1975; Regan and Beverley, 1978; Strelow and Day, 1975). Such movements were opposite to the real movements that were previously observed over an extended period of time. This may occur after looking out of railway windows for any length of time or after an abrupt halt following a long car ride, or in the form of the so-called waterfall and turntable illusions, etc. This category of apparent movements is somehow similar to successive contrasts of colours. These are consequences of selective post-excitement inhibitions of direction-sensitive movement detectors (Over, Broerse, Crassini and Lovegrove, 1973). The visual system obviously has separate lines of information for movement as well as for position in space (Regan, Beverley and Cyander, 1979). Relatively high incidences of dynamic after-images have occurred during the course of long-time presentations.

There is still a third group of dynamic after-images which may be generated by a rotating Archimedean screw. This takes the form of a shrinkage or swelling in the visual field. The same contrast of simultaneous movement may occur together with what is called the waterside phenomenon – the apparent flow towards the observer of the embankment of a flowing brook.

More apparent movements were described by Behrens and Grüsser (1977) as well as by Drischel (1961). Movements to the back or front may be also simulated by variations in size, e.g. with the projection of an image.

A phenomenon first discovered by Fertsch and first described by Pulfrich (1922) and, therefore, called the Pulfrich effect, represents apparent movements in the third dimension. An object moving in a frontal plane seems to deviate from that plane as soon as the brightness of one of the two retinal images in the observer is reduced by the application of light-absorbing glass. This may be the case if a plumb is allowed to swing over a needle. Now, if a light absorption glass is applied to the right eye, the plumb will apparently take an elliptic path to the right in front of the needle and to the left behind the needle. This is attributed to the subjective conduction time, i.e. the interval between sensory stimulation and emergence of perception conducted to the centre. As conduction time is a function of brightness, it may differ for the two eyes because of the difference in brightness. An apparent three-dimensional parallax results from the phase difference. The elliptic shape is a result of different velocities during one swing.

3. Equipment and methods for testing dynamic stereoacuity

3.1 Determination of dynamic stereoacuity

3.1.1 Binocular rotational prismometer

No method has yet been devised to determine dynamic stereoacuity. The instruments available for the measurement of monocular dynamic stereoacuity (see Section 2.1) were found to be unsuitable for testing dynamic stereoacuity unless they were enlarged by the major elements and components relating to the morphology and function of binocularity. All hardware for the determination of stereoscopy depend, for proper functionality, on a thorough exclusion of all empirical factors of three-dimensional vision (see Sections 2.3 and 2.4), which is the only way to measure the performance potential of stereoscopy proper. In this context, it has proved to be particularly difficult to avoid any influence of movement parallax by which any stereoscopic measurement would be rendered useless. This can be achieved only by ignoring the presentation of real moving test objects. Hence, the impression of test movement must be simulated. Tests based on the polarisation or anaglyph principle, have proved to be inappropriate because of the great role played by what is called stereoretardation (see Section 2.2.1), which would severely impair the output of stereoscopy as soon as the time factor became involved.

All these considerations have resulted in the invention of a binocular rotational prismometer which can be modified to meet the most specific requirements of different investigations. The apparatus can artificially generate a percept of circular movements. Yet, a minimal phenomenon similar to movement parallax may be created by eye movements alone, due to the particular position of the centre of rotation of the eye. That phenomenon, however, remains below the threshold of sensory perception and is hardly measurable by mechanical means.

The apparatus (Fig. 2) is made up of a motor with a stabiliser and set of gear wheels from which rotations are transmitted to two prism holders, each containing one prism. Centre-to-centre spacing between the two prisms is 6.4 cm, with a prism diameter of 4.5 cm. The rotational speed is directly and reliably transmitted to both prism holders so that synchronicity of rotation is safely ensured for both eyes. The rotational speed can be adjusted by a

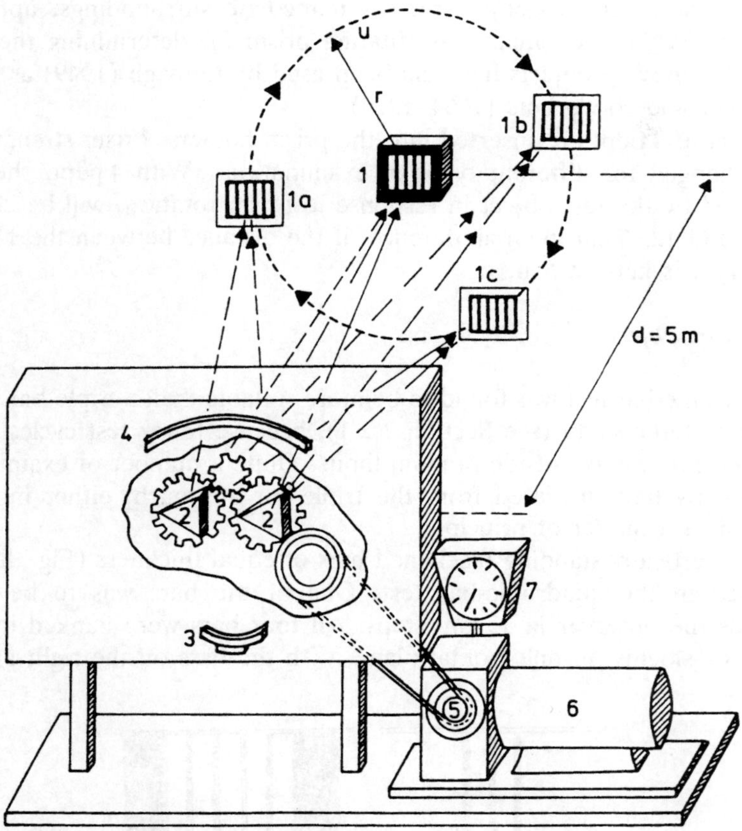

Fig. 2. Diagram of rotational prismometer (front) and quadruple-bar test (back). (1) Stereo test device with four bars; (1a–1c) Apparent movements of the test device in rotation of prisms; (2) Synchronously rotating prisms, 4 pdpt for each eye; (3) Chin rest; (4) Forehead rest; (5) Rotating disk with transmission; (6) Steplessly adjustable motor; (7) Tachometer.

transformer. Maximum prism rotation is 180 rpm. The rotational speed can be read from a calibrated tachometer. Fixed corrective lenses from a commercial spectacle lens box or a transparent sheet or blinds, may be inserted according to need in front of or behind the rotating prisms. The motor is low-noise and does not disturb the proband at all, a point which is deliberately made, since excessive noise levels may have an adverse effect on almost all variants of optosensory perception (Gramberg-Danielsen, 1976; Kitte and Dieroff, 1971; Letourneau and Milledot, 1974). A forehead bar and chin support are provided for the proband to avoid distorting head movements. The binocular field of vision is 20 angular degrees. One prism is capable of deflecting one light beam per prism diopter (pdpt) by 1 cm at a 1 m distance, which is relative to the prism base (1 pdpt = 0.57°). When the prism is allowed to rotate in front of the observer's eye, the fixed target, e.g., a test object, together with its immediate surroundings, appear to perform circular movements. A rotating prism for determining the visual acuity for moving objects had also been used by Ludvigh (1949) as well as by Jaeger and co-workers (1964–1970).

Prisms of 4 pdpt are inserted into the prism holders. Prism strengths can be exchanged for different types of examinations. With 4 pdpt, the circle described by the test object in response to prism rotation, will be 20 cm in radius and 125.7 cm in circumference, if the distance between the observer and target is kept at 5 m.

3.1.2 Test object

A quadruple-bar test was found to be more suitable than a triple-bar test for dynamic stereoacuity (see Section 2.2.1), because fewer test cycles will be required for results outside random limits. Quite a number of examiners of stereoscopy have deviated from the triple-bar approach, either in certain cases or as a matter of principle.

Four vertically standing blackened bars of equal thickness (Fig. 3b) were involved in the quadruple-bar test. One of the bars was to be moved towards the observer in 15 mm steps. All four bars were flanked by black blinds or shields, in one frontal plane, with the bars on the right and left.

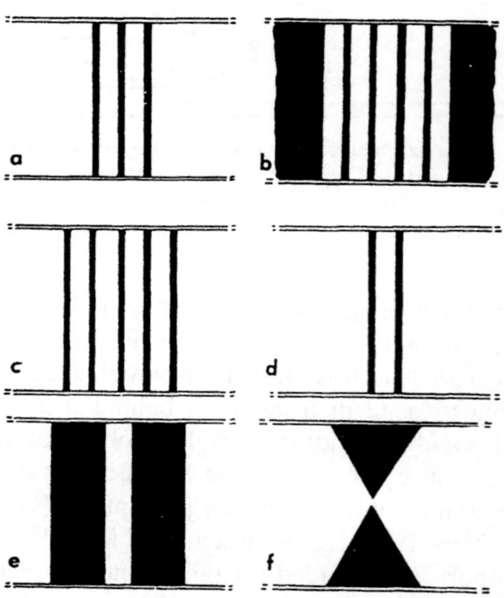

Fig. 3. Variations of triple-bar test. (a) Triple-bar apparatus; (b) Quadruple-bar apparatus of binocular rotational prismometer; (c) Five-bar apparatus (central bar to be moved forward and backward); (d) Twin-bar apparatus; (e) Cleft apparatus; (f) Double triangle according to Cords.

Table 2. Angles of disparity (in arcseconds) for all steps of the quadruple-bar test, using a rotational prismometer with a 5-metre test distance (calculated for pupillar spacings of 64 and 68 mm).

Step	Depth distance, (mm)	Lateral disparities in seconds of arc — Pupillar spacings 64 mm	68 mm
I	15	7.9″	8.4″
II	30	15.8″	16.8″
III	45	23.7″	25.2″
IV	60	31.6″	33.6″
V	75	39.6″	42.0″
VI	90	47.5″	50.4″
VII	105	55.4″	58.8″
VIII	120	63.3″	67.2″
IX	135	71.2″	75.6″
X	150	79.1″	84.0″

Lateral disparity for all adjustable steps may be seen from Table 2, as calculated by the Helmholtz' formula $p = at/d^2 \times 206{,}000$ (p = binocular position parallax in arc seconds; a = pupillar spacing in mm; t = real depth distance in mm; d = test distance in mm).

The influence of pupillar spacing (a) has proved to be of only minor importance and, therefore, can be neglected without any risk (Table 2). Maximum deviations likely to result from neglecting pupillar spacing were found to be ±10 percent for the measurement of small stereoacuity values. Normal stereoacuity measured by this apparatus was found to be somewhere between 8 and 40 arcseconds, which, for a 5 m distance, would mean a real depth distance of 15–75 mm.

Four adjustments are possible with each test problem or each depth distance for the quadruple-bar test, in conjunction with other modern monocular and binocular vision tests (Landolt rings, Pflüger hooks, Titmus tests, Randot tests, TNO tests, Pola tests, children optotypes, etc.). One of the four bars is moved out of the frontal plane and must be identified by the person being tested. The bars can only be moved in a forward direction. This is a limitation that is in keeping with all modern stereotests. Polarisation and anaglyphic tests, too, are restricted to cross-over lateral disparity, i.e. forward readjustment of one in four test figures. Testing of dynamic stereoacuity is characterised by an additional peculiarity that only forward movement has any relevance to visual perception in everyday life and occupational practice. Adjustments can be both forward and backward with the classical triple-bar apparatus. Centre-to-centre bar spacing is 14.5 mm throughout (=10′ visual angle). The spacings can be widened up to 87 mm (=60′). The thickness of each bar is 3.6 mm (=2.5′ visual angle) (see Section 5.1.2). The blackened bars are kept in front of a white wall which is *ca.*

620 cd/m^2 in luminance. Ambient luminance in the test room was *ca.* 150 cd/m^2. These conditions satisfied the relatively stringent international demands on lighting for vision testing. According to these specifications (Aulhorn, 1976; Schober, 1976), test-field luminance should be between 150 and 670 cd/m^2 in the immediate vicinity of the optotype (background of the bars for the quadruple-bar test). The luminance of the optotype (bars and blinds for the quadruple-bar test) should account for no more than 10 percent of the test-field luminance. These conditions are normally met by the quadruple-bar test, since the bars are deep-black and not translucent and glossy. Luminance for visual angles between 10 and 25 degrees should be reduced to 25 percent of the test field luminance, but should never be allowed to drop below 10 percent at any point. Glare effects must be avoided.

Polarisation and anaglyphic tests have quite often been used on static testing because of their convenient handling. Their applications may also appear to be tempting in the testing of dynamic stereoscopy. However, luminance and contrast have so far been unsatisfactory in almost all instances. Also, polarisation and anaglyphic procedures are based on a relatively unnatural experimental arrangement. Their use is restricted to testing the sensory capability of translating lateral disparate retinal percepts into three-dimensional perceptions, without the totality of all aspects important to three-dimensional vision being involved (Mehlhose, 1975). Random dot stereograms can also be used for testing dynamic stereoacuity, using two projectors and rectangularly crossed polarisation. However, as random dot stereograms provide non-contoured test images, stereoretardation (see Section 2.2.2) would be greatly extended in moving-object vision tests, and additional problems would crop up in connection with fusion. Both stereoretardation and fusion-related problems were found to have severely adverse effects upon test results.

The binocular rotational prismometer and the quadruple-bar test are also suitable for routine investigations. It is a great additional physiologico-optical advantage of both that the test field in constant extension and unchanged content, consistently stays within the field of vision. This is likely to eliminate the problems of movement-related brightness variation and adaptation. Also, the test remains within the field of view instead of emerging, time and again, in the periphery, as usually happens, when horizontal movements are tested by means of reflector systems.

3.1.3 Testing method

The examination of a person being tested is preceded by a thorough briefing on the purpose and task of the test. This is usually followed by preparatory exercises, including about 10 adjustments. Ludvigh and Miller (1958) found that this number was sufficient to eliminate 90 percent of all possible effects of individual human factors relating to dynamic visual acuity (see Section 2.1). Short breaks are intercalated after some 20 adjustments to avoid fatigue. A somewhat extended break is inserted as soon as fatigue symptoms become obvious through complaints by probands or a deterioration of test results. Any testing should be preceded by an examination of the vision of the person tested. Test parameters have to be verified after long intervals to ensure constant test conditions. Bishop (1975) suggested that stereoacuity depended much more on variations in contrast and room lighting than did ordinary visual acuity.

During the test, one of the four bars is pulled forward, beginning with the highest adjustable depth distance of 150 mm = 79.1″. The test begins with the setting of a high rotational speed which is then gradually reduced until the bar positions can be recognised. Four adjustments are arithmetically averaged. Six to eight adjustments will have to be made in the case of too large a discrepancy between individual results. All the average values of these adjustments should be plotted into a diagram, with its abscissa giving the stereoacuity in arcseconds (lateral disparity) or real depth distance in millimeters, and its ordinate given in rpm values or path in degrees per second.

The number of rotations (rpm) should always be converted to degrees per second (°/sec) for a better comparison of current test results and those recorded for dynamic visual acuity by earlier examiners (Miller and Ludvigh, 1958). Primarily, this would require a calculation of the length of the circular orbit described by the test in response to a defined prism strength and number of angular degrees. Then the path of one arc degree travelled by a test object in a 5 m viewing distance is determined, and the length of the rotation has to be divided by that path value. The result will show the number of angular degrees of an apparent circular orbit of the tests in response to one single prism rotation, related to the viewing distance. The path (in degrees travelled per second) will be obtained by dividing the viewing distance by the number of seconds required for one circular orbit.

Stereoscopic percepts take only a fraction of a second to achieve optimum sensory performance (Monje, 1969). After all, a moving object is fixed by the eye some four to five times per second (Söllner, 1961). A much longer time is required for a single readjustment and for an individual test using the binocular rotational prismometer, because a reduction of initial speed for the recognition of depth-distance must be made slowly (roughly 10 sec per step). Time is not usually considered in the testing of static stereoacuity, although it is generally known that staring at an object for a long time will lead to poor test results. Hence, there is a greater risk of fatigue and a decrease in attention and interest.

The fact that quite a number of examiners only tested between three and ten persons for their studies into dynamic visual acuity, may be attributable to the time-consuming nature of dynamic function testing. The time needed for testing dynamic stereoacuity has proved to be 10 times greater than that required for dynamic visual acuity testing. This is because four to six optotypes may be simultaneously presented in dynamic visual acuity tests, whereas only one test position can be set for any single dynamic stereoacuity test, which takes much more time than the exchange of optotypes for the projection of a series.

A too-lengthy presentation time is just as undesirable as one that is too short. A too long fixation was found to cause a flattening in space, often referred to as the 'Lilliputian effect' (Ebbecke, 1948). The same flattening phenomenon was recorded as a consequence of a local adaptation from static stereoscopy testing by von Helmholtz and Hering. This phenomenon was found to cause miscalculations of distance and velocity by car drivers after a long time on the road.

It would be extremely useful to obtain all results of dynamic stereoacuity objectivated by VECP recordings. Yet, attempts made so far, in that direction have not been very successful. True, efforts have been made using VECP to determine the presence of stereoscopy and stereoacuity (Vomberg and Skrandies, 1985). However, random dot chessboard patterns have been used in all these investigations, and here, if VECP is used, the best achievable values for stereoscopy are much higher than those recordable from natural tests and from the subjective information provided by probands exposed, for example, to the triple-bar apparatus. No stereoscopy was recordable from a significant number of normally sighted probands tested with random dot patterns. Also, the dot patterns were relatively general in polarisation-haploscopic reflector systems with two monitors. The luminance values used, about 3 cd/m^2 (see Section 4.1), proved to be insufficient for practice-relevant investigations, since they came very close to twilight vision. Such results are not yet satisfactory enough to be used for any judgement on road traffic and working conditions.

3.2 Determination of kinetoparallactic stereoacuity

3.2.1 Parallactoscopometer

All systems and hardware described in the literature for determining threshold values in dynamic parallactoscopy were invented prior to 1940 and are burdened with severe drawbacks and shortcomings, when measured by today's standards. Cords (1913) and von Tschermak (1938) dealt with dynamic parallactoscopy when working on expert opinions, but their attention was confined to the active variant (head motion). Obviously, passive dynamic parallactoscopy, had never been investigated in relation to cases of moving visual objects, although it should have been of some interest for occupational medicine.

Hence, studies into dynamic parallactoscopy called for the development of a new apparatus with which to measure monocular stereoacuity for moving objects on the basis of movement parallax. This was to be called a 'parallactoscopometer' although its name would not betray its dual purpose – the assessment of both active and passive dynamic parallactoscopy. The test object can be moved at various speeds, and the use of a variety of different test figures is also possible.

Major consideration was given to practice-related aspects in the development of the new apparatus. A variable-width shield was attached to the front. Behind this, a carriage for the test object was placed which could be moved to and fro over 0.8 m (Fig. 4). The test carriage was pulled by a driving tongue in an endless gearwheel chain which was connected to a motor by a belt. The motor speed was steplessly varied by modification of the tension. Four measuring sensors were provided to generate a current impulse, as soon as they came into contact with the test carriage, for high-accuracy control of the carriage travelling time and constant speed. Several relays were provided for limit switching and automatic change-over to different speeds or motor outputs, the latter being of particular importance for non-horizontal movements. The motor, to which two alternatively

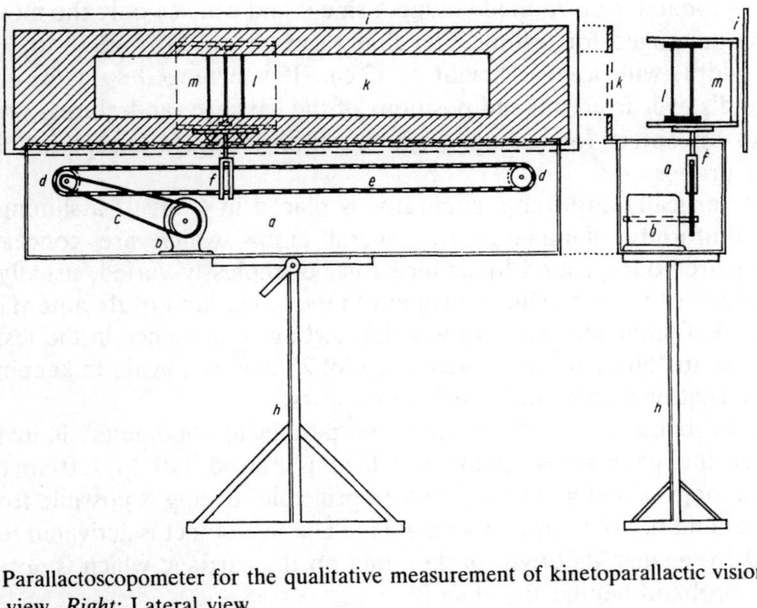

Fig. 4. Parallactoscopometer for the qualitative measurement of kinetoparallactic vision. *Left:* Frontal view. *Right:* Lateral view.

(*a*) Casing (front cover removed) with motor and chain drive for travelling test carriage; (*b*) Motor; (*c*) Transmission belt; (*d*) Geared wheels; (*e*) Gear wheel chain; (*f*) Driving tongue for test carriage with pin, the latter moving to and fro in a slit of the upper casing; (*g*) Shaft for apparatus inclination; (*h*) Apparatus frame; (*i*) White rear screen; (*k*) Window through front stage (hatched) covering upper and lower fixtures of test figure and test carriage; (*l*) Triple-bar test; (*m*) Movable carriage with test figure.

applicable and steplessly adjustable transformers are connected, is actually the centerpiece of the functional component. For horizontal operation, the carriage speed can be steplessly varied between 0.12 and 1 m/s. A control apparatus with an electromechanical stop-watch is provided for determining the real object speed. It may be used for time measurements from 100 milliseconds to 24 hours at a measuring accuracy of ±10 milliseconds. It may also be used for automatic change-over via relays or for disconnection, say, when certain typical situations, according to variable preset programmes, are scanned by the four measuring sensors.

The drive mechanism is accommodated in a light metal casing. The functional component can be raised to eye level along a steel tube holder. Its dimensions are 125 cm in length, 26 cm in width, and 22 cm in height plus another 28 cm to allow for the shield level in front of the moving carriage. The holder is strong enough to keep the apparatus stable, even at high-speed operation. This enables the functional component to rotate by 90 degrees to either side, thus, allowing testing with object movement in horizontal, diagonal, and vertical directions. The testing carriage has a base which is 12 cm in length and 10 cm in width and can travel to and fro on guide rails. A frame can be attached to it by means of thumb screws to hold easily interchangeable test objects.

The proband is positioned behind a shield and can see only the movement section envisaged for testing. The shield can be varied from 10 to 80 cm in clear width, with a clear height of 12 cm. It is arranged so as to hide the proband's eyes from the end positions of the carriage, and, during presentation of an object for testing, from the entire carriage except for the test object proper.

The vertically adjustable apparatus is placed in front of a shining white wall, uniformly illuminated by several lamps which are concealed to avoid glare. Background luminance can be steplessly varied, usually up to 620 cd/m^2, which is a value equivalent to the lower limit of the internationally specified luminance values for vision testing. Luminance in the test room was close to 150 cd/m^2 at a visual angle of 25 degrees, again in keeping with the international rules for visual acuity tests.

The proband, seated 4.5 m from the parallactoscopometer, is invited to look at the parallactoscopometer which is placed 110 to 130 cm off the ground, approximately at eye level. In principle, testing is possible from any distance and not only from above 4.5 m. The test object is activated to move to and fro against its bright background on the carriage which is not visible to the proband behind the shield.

One of the proband's eyes is covered for testing to enable only monocular vision, even in cases of intact binocular vision. For determination of passive parallactoscopy, the proband's head must be additionally fixed by means of a combination of chin and forehead rests. Such examination conditions are imposed on the proband to render almost ineffective all secondary empirical possibilities for space judgement (see Section 2.4), except for dynamic parallactoscopy, which is the subject of testing. No role is played by either convergence or accommodation due to the low depth differences.

Selection for tests of the above kind was limited to individuals with a visual acuity of at least 0.4 diopters and a maximum spectacle lens correction of ±2 diopters (including astigmatism up to 1 diopters) of the eye that had to be examined. All testing was monocular.

3.2.2 Test object

The triple-bar test (see Section 2.2.1) was used as the test object. It was originally invented for measuring binocular depth acuity and is still used for that purpose. However, it also proved to be suitable as a test figure for the parallactoscopometer and provides the additional advantage of convenient comparability with the much greater number of results recorded from earlier examinations of depth acuity (=stereoacuity).

The bars used in testing were 3.6 mm in thickness, with a visible length of 12 cm (Fig. 3). Their mid-point spacing was 15 or 5 mm, so that the visual angle of observation amounted to 11′28″ from a test distance of 4.5 m. The central bar could be moved forward and backward in 15 mm steps, up to 120 mm in either direction (=480″ kinetoparallactic stereoacuity). Yet, the depth-distance of bars, measured in mm, was of no great relevance, as the testing distance was not considered. It would be better to specify the depth-distance of the bars in percentages in relation to test distance (relative depth difference; Table 3a). The relative depth difference can be calculated with any angle of observation (in angular seconds, ″) from the given kinetoparallactoscopic threshold value and independent of distance. Such calculations can be made by the Helmholtz formula for the determination of binocular depth acuity (see Section 2.2.2).

Table 3a. Conversion of threshold values measured in mm (real depth distances) on triple-bar apparatus of a parallactoscopometer to percentages of test distance and angular seconds for an observation line of 40 cm and a test distance of 4.5 m.

Real depth distances (mm)	Depth distances converted to percent of test distance (4.5 m) (%)	Depth distances converted to angular seconds (″)
120	2.66	480
105	2.33	420
90	2.00	360
75	1.66	300
60	1.33	240
45	1.00	180
30	0.66	120
15	0.33	60

The following simplified formula can be used with the parallactoscopometer for the calculation of stereoacuity at observation angles below 10 degrees:

$$S \approx 36 \cdot \alpha \cdot \frac{d}{a},$$

where S (″) stands for stereoacuity, d (cm) for depth difference, a (m) for average observation distance, and α for the angle of observation. Hence, the values given in Table 3b would apply for a test distance of 4.5 m.

To indicate individual kinetoparallactic vision performance, it does not make any difference if the proband is moving (active kinetoparallactoscopy) or if a relative movement takes place between probands/observer and depth-different visual objects (passive kinetoparallactoscopy) (Fig. 5).

3.2.3 *Testing method*

Testing of visual acuity is followed by qualitative determination of active kinetoparallactoscopy. This is started by the triple-bar test of the stopped carriage of the parallactoscopometer at a test distance of 4.5 m. The proband is permitted to carry out head and body movements up to five times at any intensity or speed, in a seated position and with a maximum width of 40 cm (movement parallax). The preselected test problem will be recorded as unresolved if more than five are made. Experience has proved that more than five movements do not lead to major improvements in the results.

The head of the proband has to be fixed by means of a combined chin and forehead rest for subsequent testing of passive parallactoscopy. The carriage along with the test object is moved in frontoparallel direction relative to the patient at a predetermined speed of 0.5 m/s (see Section 5.2.5), with one movement being made in either direction within a visible observation line of 40 cm. Hence, the test object can be observed by the proband for 0.8 seconds with an angular velocity of 6.3 °/sec. Variation of velocity can be ignored, since no substantial difference would be shown by dynamic paral-

Table 3b. Stereoacuity (″) on the basis of kinetoparallactoscopy, depending on the observation angle (α) and relative depth difference (d/a), with indications of observation line and depth difference for selected test distance ($a = 4.5$ m).

Relative depth difference (d/a) (%)	Depth differences (d) for $a = 4.5$ m (mm)	Observation angles of lines for $a = 4.5$ m (″)			
		1° 8 cm	2° 16 cm	5° 40 cm	10° 80 cm
0.33	15	12	24	60	120
0.66	30	24	48	120	240
1.0	45	36	72	180	360
2.0	90	72	144	360	720

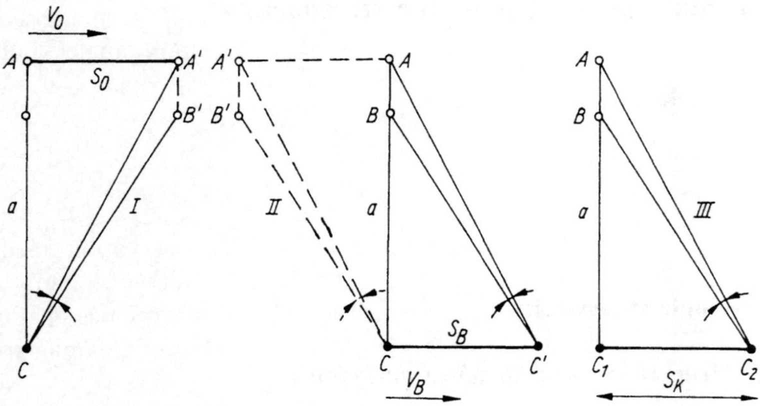

Fig. 5. Geometrical conditions for dynamic parallactoscopy. *a:* Object of observation. A and B are two depth-distant objects, C the observer's eye.
I: Passive parallactoscopy (movement of depth-distant objects A and B to A′ and B′); V_0 object velocity; ACA′ viewing angle or necessary ocular pursuit movement; A′CB′ angle of parallactic shift; S_0 viewing path of objects A and B.
II: Passive movement of the observer's eye. S_B distance passed by the observer's eye within a given observation time; V_B observer's velocity; S pathway of apparent object movement; AC′B angle of parallactic shift.
III: Active parallactoscopy, with head or body movement. S_k extent of head or body movements (basis of parallactic shift); C_1AC_2 viewing angle; AC_2B angle of parallactic shift.

lactoscopy with the velocities preset on the parallactoscopometer (0.12 to 1 m/s).

Testing is started at the largest test distance adjustable on the apparatus (120 mm), with adjustments being made forward and backward. Subsequent adjustments are made unsystematically in the forward and back directions. The next largest depth distance is chosen after five correct answers in succession, with the steps being 30 mm at the beginning, 15 mm from the depth distance at 60 mm, and 5 mm from a depth distance below 30 mm.

The test commences with the introduction or initiation of five to 10 test positions to allow for any forthcoming test effects. The average test is 10 minutes per proband. Three or four short breaks are intercalated to avoid fatigue or loss of attention, the lengths of such breaks being specified according to individual requirements. Testing for kinetoparallactoscopy has proved to require much more time than testing for dynamic stereoacuity, since at least five different adjustments or settings of the apparatus are necessary for each step.

The proband is required to choose between the position of the central bar being in front of the two lateral bars or behind. The same arrangement regarding depth distance is presented to the proband at least five times in irregular order of 'in front' or 'behind'. Identification of the adjusted depth difference can be concluded with an error probability of 5 percent, if all the answers are correct. The proband is allowed to make one mistake for a 'correct' rating in tests with seven different settings.

4. Normal values of dynamic stereoacuity

4.1 Dynamic stereoacuity

4.1.1 *Mean values and standard deviation*

Tests using the rotational prismometer were applied to 103 normally sighted persons being tested to elucidate the relationship between dynamic stereoacuity and velocity of movement. Static stereoacuity was 16″ transverse disparation or better in all probands. Mean values and standard deviations recorded from that mass screening are given in Fig. 6. A coordinate system with curve ascension to the right has been used in this illustration to allow for the idea that growing rotational speed is accompanied by an increase in actually identified depth distance, i.e. size of

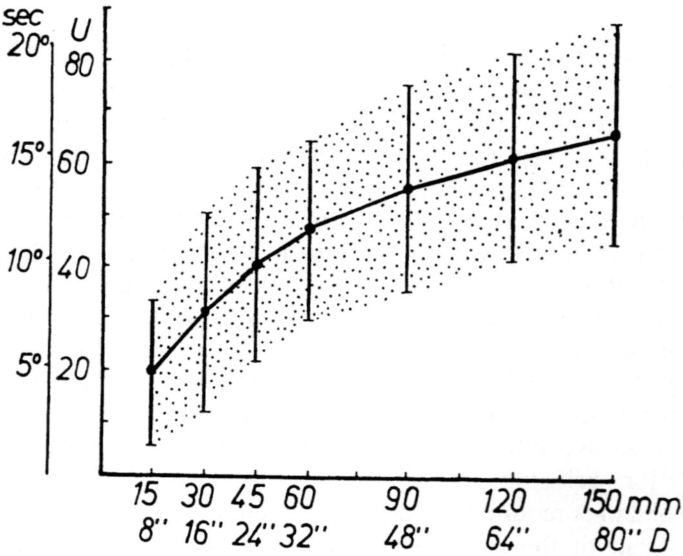

Fig. 6. Mean values and standard deviation of dynamic stereoacuity ($n = 103$), as determined by rotational prismometer (circular movements) and quadruple-bar test. Abscissa: Depth distance of bars (mm), and as angle of lateral disparity (*D*) in angular seconds (″). Ordinate: Revolutions per minute (right) and path in degrees per second (°/sec).

transverse disparation. However, in this context, one would have to put up with the fact that the direction of curve plotting is contrary to the course of testing, since any testing would be started with the high transverse disparations which, in the system of coordinates, are plotted to the abscissa on the right. Mean-value curves correspond to the common picture of optosensory perception: finer steps of sensory performance are much more susceptible to stress factors than general steps with lower demands on vision.

All probands suggested that the stereoscopic impression they had with a still target was not impaired by slow movement of the test figure. A few probands even reported that stereoscopic vision was enhanced or, at least, facilitated by slow movement of the test figure. This, however, could not be confirmed by measurement, as long as the step method was used. No improved vision in response to slow optotype movement was recorded either by Jaeger and Honegger (1964) in their measurements of monocular dynamic visual acuity and was not even recorded by them from Snellen's near vision charts with their relatively subtle graduation. A measurable improvement of vision, similar to the findings reported by Söllner (1961), was recorded only by Schober, Junker and Grimm (1967) who had used a special (sliding) method on three test persons. Those findings were made up to 5 °/s. However, the improvement of visual acuity recorded by them was relatively low and differed greatly among individuals. Improvement of visual acuity in ocular pursuit of slowly moving optotypes has been attributed to avoidance or reduction of local adaptation which would necessarily occur along with continuous watching of an object (see Section 2.1).

The question remains to be answered as to why dynamic stereoacuity tends to decrease relatively soon along with growing velocity, although the human eye is capable of extremely rapid movement and although only a fraction of a second is needed for stereoscopic perception. Also, very little time is required for response, i.e. to catch a visual object by ocular pursuit and saccadic eye movements. The decline in visual performance is attributable to the relatively inadequate mechanism of binocular fixation. Object movements correspond to ocular pursuit movements only in slow-movement tests (Honegger, 1970). Even very slight acceleration will entail a continuous decline in ocular pursuit accuracy, resulting in larger corrective jumps until the moving target can no longer be recognised, ending any eye movement. With medium velocities, sensory evaluation of a visual impression will be satisfactory only if the mechanism of fixation proves to be capable of keeping the target fixated for some time within the central or paracentral area of fixation. Dynamic stereoacuity tends to drop, when the visual object is perceived more and more by peripheral points of the retina, just as in the case of dynamic visual acuity. The standard deviation in the context of dynamic stereoacuity was found to be very much higher than that recordable from elementary static visual acuity. This proved to be basically attributable to a multitude of factors which, in different probands, had differentiated effects on stereoscopic vision (see Section 2.2.2) and on vision of moving targets, not to mention variations in attention and interest. As suggested by the sensory physiologist Monje (1969), any perception of moving objects may be affected by slight changes of luminance, adaptation, and formation of the after-image.

The enormous scatter of test results, even in the context of monocular visual acuity, has been underlined by Ludvigh (1949). That was one of the conspicuous findings obtained from 1,000 naval aviator cadets reported by Ludvigh and Miller (1958), although this group of probands had been relatively homogeneous with regard to sex, intelligence, exposure to demand, fatigue, and age. The scatter was so large that the probands were subdivided by three groups for easier overseeability: (1) a group in which velocity had considerable impact upon monocular visual acuity, (2) a group in which movement had surprisingly little influence upon visual acuity, and (3) a group with transitional phenomena.

A distinction could easily be made among different behaviours for dynamic stereoacuity, as well. All probands with above-average dynamic stereoacuity in response to considerable velocities of movement did not exhibit good dynamic stereoacuity in response to low velocities. Opposite behaviours were not rare either.

Typical behaviour of probands, together with their percentual representation in the overall group, are illustrated in Fig. 7. Only 10 percent of all test

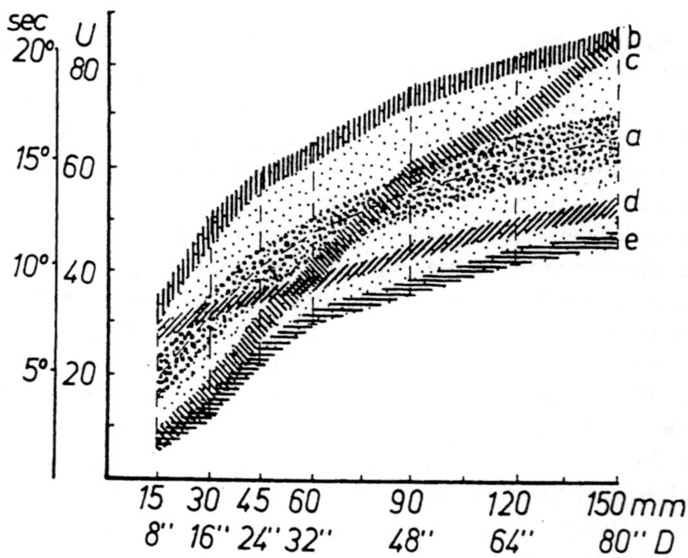

Fig. 7. Typical reactions of dynamic stereoacuity ($n = 103$) to rpm variations. Percentual values for various types of behaviour, relative to total group: (*a*) 40%; (*b*) 16%; (*c*) 8%; (*d*) 12%; (*e*) 14%. Ten percent of probands were not classifiable because they did not fit in with the above pattern. Abscissa and ordinate as in Fig. 6.

persons could not be associated with any of the three categories for their stereoscopic vision. Prediction of a category to which a test person should be linked is generally impossible on the basis of one single measurement of dynamic stereoacuity.

There is no normal distribution of measuring results. Ludvigh and Miller (1958) tried to derive the following formula from their own curves of monocular dynamic visual acuity:

$$y = \alpha + b \cdot x^3 .$$

The curve of dynamic stereoacuity is like a parabola, with a steep initial rise being followed by a gradual deceleration of that rise which is approximate to a horizontal. It may be expressed by the following equation:

$$y = \alpha + b_1 x + b_2 x^2 + b_3 x^3 ,$$

where a = regression constant; b_1, b_2, and b_3 = regression coefficients; y = number of revolutions; x = depth distance in mm.

Flattening of the curve in response to higher velocities should primarily be attributed to the effects of secondary (empirical) factors of three-dimensional perception, especially in connection with size comparison. For example, a bar moved forward through an adjustment of the binocular rotational prismometer to the maximum of 150 mm, would appear to be 3 percent wider than it is in reality when viewed from a distance of 5 m. All empirical factors of three-dimensional perception (see Sections 2.3 and 2.4) are much more stable than stereoscopy regarding effects of movement vision, and in response to a continuous increase of velocity, they are capable of eventually replacing or eliminating stereoscopy (see Section 8).

4.1.2 Effect of age

Roughly 10,000 million cells exist in the human brain at the time of birth and tend to undergo a sizeable shooting of their neuraxons or nerve processes during childhood and adolescence, resulting in the propagation of synaptic connections and a growing capability of association. The number of cells then will gradually begin to drop above the age of 45 years, which at first can be sufficiently compensated by experience, exercise, and effort but will gradually lead to a decrease in general fitness and performance, not to mention possible pathological processes. These developments are relevant to involvement in road traffic. The man-vehicle-road complex may be considered a control circuit (Lücking and Struppler, 1982) in which the sensory organs have to pick up information. It is the sensory organs' age-dependent translation into reactions which will substantially determine a driver's conduct on the road. True, increasing age generally goes together with an overestimation of one's own efficiency but, on the other hand, is accompanied by overcautiousness, higher rating of safety, and decreasing inclination towards taking risks (Höllen-Hubert, Aigner and Kastenhuber, 1975; Kroj, 1972). This is the reason why the accident rate involving drivers of advanced age is lower than that of younger drivers, except for professional drivers (Sanders, 1970). Driving fitness generally declines with growing age (Gramberg-Danielsen, 1967).

Contradictory data have been published in the literature about the effect of age on stereoscopic threshold vision. No effects of age were recorded by some more recent authors (Hofstetter and Bertsch, 1976; Linschotten, 1956; Römhild, 1983; Vokes, 1980). Opposite findings have usually been attributable to differences in vision, since visual acuities between 1.25 and 1.5 are much more frequent in younger individuals than in higher age, although the lower visual acuity of people of advanced age is not usually considered for statistical evaluation of mass screening. At higher age levels, even vision of 0.7 is quite often rated as normal.

Honegger, Schaefer and Jaeger (1969) compared the values of monocular dynamic visual acuity of normally sighted persons aged between 20 and 30 years with those recorded from probands aged between 50 and 60 years and found that persons of advanced age showed results that were clearly worse than those of younger people. Similar findings were recorded by Burg (1964, 1966). They were presumably not only associated with the delayed reactivity of aged persons but were even more so attributable to a loss of accuracy in sensorial oculomotoricity. According to Piper (1969), growing age is accompanied by the degradation of oculomotoricity, so that ocular adjustments in the paracentral and peripheral fields of vision are delayed and are likely to become less accurate. This, however, would be of particular importance to ocular pursuit of moving objects. Limited mobility of the cervical spine in individuals of advanced age can be neglected in this context, since the results were the same for both fixed and freely mobile heads.

The assumption, therefore, can be made that dynamic stereoacuity also becomes reduced at higher age. Individuals below the age of 40 were compared to those above, with the younger probands providing significantly better results, the error probability being 0.1 percent.

4.1.3 Effect of sex

Several examiners have tried unsuccessfully to discover if there are sex-related differences in static stereoacuity (depth acuity). A literature review on the subject was compiled by Linschotten (1956). No sex-related differences were recorded by Römhild (1983) in her studies into static depth acuity using the triple-bar apparatus. Differences should be expected, since the average pupil distances of women and, consequently, their positional parallax, are smaller than those of men. For example, with a test distance of

5 m, a depth distance of 10 mm with a positional parallax (=pupillary distance) of 60 mm would give a transverse disparation of 4.9″, but with a positional parallax of 65 mm, the transverse disparation should be 5.4″. In other words, persons who, by virtue of their physiology, have a smaller average pupillary distance, above all women and children, should be somewhat inferior in stereoacuity to individuals with wider pupillary distance. In relation to this context, it was pointed out by Blasius (1953) that the average stereoscopic vision of individuals alerted to colour is worse than that of individuals oriented to shape. Women, as a matter of fact, are more commonly colour-oriented than men.

The 103 probands included 63 women and 40 men. Statistical calculation did not reveal any significant difference between the two groups.

4.1.4 Effect of occupational activity

Occupational effects on dynamic stereoacuity might be possible under the following two aspects. An occupational activity permanently calling for high dynamic stereoacuity might lead to a specific improvement in performance due to practice. Yet, it is also possible that occupations with high demands on dynamic stereoacuity are primarily chosen by individuals whose excellent dynamic stereoacuity had previously been established. With regard to static stereoscopy, the first aspect has been denied by the majority of authors. Cases which revealed an apparent relationship between occupation and stereoacuity were probably attributable to the pre-existence of higher stereoacuity. The second aspect has been analysed Römhild (1983), especially after the average static stereoacuity she had recorded in a mass screening programme of individuals involved in stereoscopic evaluation in cartography and geodesy, had proved to be significantly better than values recorded from other persons. A certain amount of selection, of course, cannot be ruled out, since persons with moderate to poor stereoacuity will soon abandon or be forced to abandon employment with high demands on stereoscopic vision because of optosensory insufficiency.

Occupational groups do not differ from each other for dynamic stereoacuity, although none of the 103 test persons was occupationally exposed to particular demands on static and dynamic stereoscopy. It is, therefore, absolutely possible that persons with insufficient dynamic stereoacuity cannot continue indefinitely in occupations which depend on high performance in dynamic vision.

4.1.5 Comparison between dynamic stereoacuity and dynamic visual acuity

It is very tempting to make a comparison between results obtained from dynamic visual acuity testing on the one hand and those of dynamic stereoacuity testing on the other. Problems of doing so are implied in the different structures of both sensory functions. Visual acuity is of an elementary nature and is relatively independent, whereas the existence of stereoacuity would not be possible without visual acuity which is mainly a function of the foveal cells of the retina. Dynamic stereoacuity is based on the functional systems in the visual cortex, representing a highly complex associative achievement of the central nervous system with many aspects depending on it. Growing velocity and consecutive decline in visual performance down to a level at which gaze movements can no longer pursue a moving target, are not the primary causes for limitation of performance, since the human eye is capable of moving at about 500 °/s, with velocities of even 260 °/s having been recorded from dynamic visual acuity tests (Miller and Ludvigh, 1962).

The insufficiency of the sensomotor mechanism of fixation is the decisive cause underlying a given performance in response to growing velocity in both dynamic visual acuity and dynamic stereoacuity. Lines of tracking or pursuit of ocular movements tend to become less accurate as velocity is increased, and the test object cannot be held sufficiently long within the area of fixation. It gradually becomes projected to those retinal areas with resolution powers which are insufficient for adequate visual recognition or identification. It is because of such an inadequate fixation capability that dynamic visual acuity for circular movements is four times worse than that for horizontal movements (Ludvigh, 1949) when the same angular velocity is provided. This point has been *additionally* supported by the results recorded so far from dynamic visual acuity testing of old and young probands. The differences in precise fixation are considerable. Erratic movements of fixation, no doubt, are a consequence of the limits to the central association of optomotoricity and optosensoricity (Drischel, 1961).

The method and arrangements chosen for the tests of dynamic visual acuity described below were identical with those used in dynamic stereoacuity testing, although the quadruple-bar test was replaced by optotypes (Pflüger's hooks) of the acuity projector supplied from Carl Zeiss Jena. For a more convenient comparison with binocular stereoacuity, dynamic visual acuity was binocularly tested. This proved to be practicable, and without any problems, with the binocular rotational prismometer. Ten of 13 normally sighted probands exhibited a static binocular vision of 1.25, with as much as 1.5 having been recorded from four of them.

The results recorded from this experimental series, together with mean-value curve and standard deviation, were included in the same diagram as the findings obtained from a mass screening for dynamic stereoacuity (Fig. 8). It was, however, a problem coordinating the curve of dynamic visual acuity with that of dynamic stereoacuity. This proved only to be feasible in the sense of approximation. Stereoacuity of 15 mm in depth distance was equalled to a binocular vision acuity of *ca*. 1.25. A depth distance of 150 mm consequently represented a stereoscopic vision of 10 percent (0.1). Never-

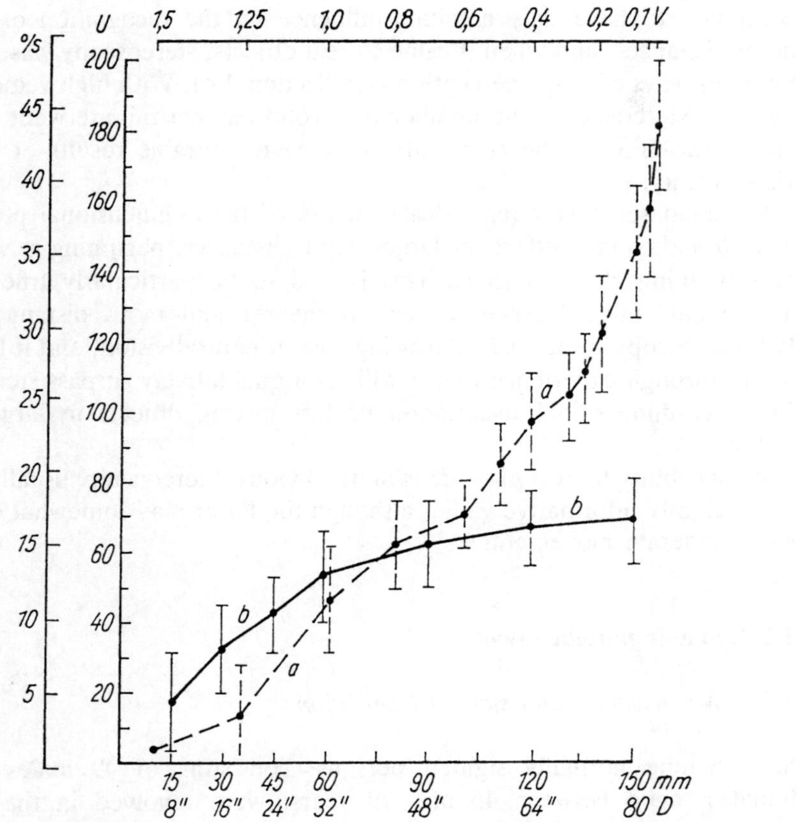

Fig. 8. Comparison of dynamic visual acuity thresholds (visual acuity for moving objects) (*a*) and dynamic stereoacuity (*b*). Abscissa below: Depth distance of bars (mm), and as angle of lateral disparity (*D*). Abscissa top: Visual acuity (*V*) in decimal values, from 1.5 to 0.04. Ordinate: Revolutions per minute (right) and path in degrees per second (left).

theless, the characteristic differences in either curve were quite conspicuous within one and the same system of coordinates, even without diagram composition.

Basic differences were found to exist between the two curves, irrespective of their form of representation. The curve for dynamic visual acuity was slowly but steadily rising in response to low velocities, the rise clearly getting steeper along with increasing velocities, so that total insufficiency could be expected at high velocities, e.g., above 200 rpm. None of the probands exhibited a vision of 0.04 at a velocity of 200 rpm. The values established for dynamic visual acuity were almost completely identical with those reported by Jaeger and Honegger (1958). The curve for dynamic stereoacuity, on the other hand, tended to rise rapidly at the beginning along with a growing velocity, and was soon to be followed by transition to an almost horizontal orientation with only slight ascension. In other words, high velocities continued to have only a minor influence on the recognition of general depth distances, and when it came to real objects, stereoscopy was replaced by other ways of space perception (see Section 2.4). With high velocities for dynamic stereoacuity, the number of revolutions per minute went down to about one-third of the rpm still providing measurable results of dynamic visual acuity.

So-called secondary (empirical) factors of three-dimensional perception were found to take effect for larger-depth distances, beginning at velocities of something close to 15 °/s. This is said to be particularly true for the assessment, by difference in size, of nearer and more distant objects. Parallactoscopy, too, plays a growing role in natural vision, and it has been found through experience that it will soon qualitatively surpass stereoscopy for three-dimensional localisation of fast-moving objects in larger-depth distances.

Applicability to everyday life is quite obvious. Stereoacuity usually retains a sufficiently informative value, although the latter may somewhat decrease with moderate movements.

4.2 Dynamic parallactoscopy

4.2.1 Mean values and standard deviation

Seventy-nine normally sighted persons, consisting of 49 males and 30 females, aged between 15 and 79 years, were involved in the routine examinations described. The average age was 39.5 years (standard deviation being ±16.5 years). The mean value of the reference visual acuity was 0.86 (standard deviation: 0.19). Right-eye predominance was slightly pronounced among the probands, the right-left ratio being 41:38. Age, sex, side of tested eye, visual acuity, and vocational background were recorded from all probands. The better or more healthy eye was used for monocular testing in all cases, with the other eye occasionally being blindfolded.

Parallactoscopy was determined with active movement (head and body movements) using the triple-bar test, and with passive movement it was determined by moving the test figure on the parallactoscopometer (see Section 3.2.3).

Dynamic parallactoscopy with head and body movements, quite often unintentionally used for three-dimensional perception, gave a mean value for the still-detectable space difference with the parallactoscopometer at a test distance of 4.5 m (2.7 cm), which was equivalent to a parallactoscopic stereoacuity of 108″ (see Section 3.2.3). There was no normal distribution, as is the case in almost all optosensorial threshold determinations. The frequency distribution thus established is given in Fig. 9. The values which were rated normal, sufficient, pathological, or insufficient with regard to

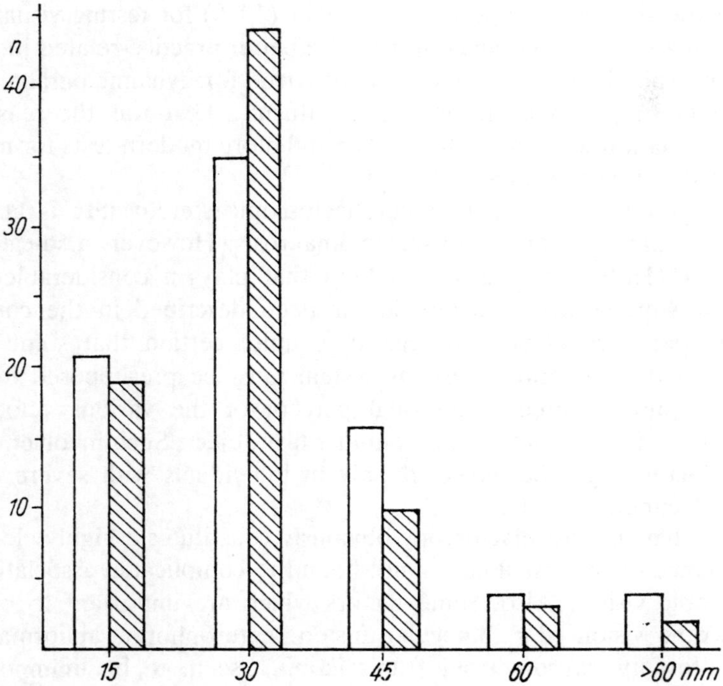

Fig. 9. Frequency of stereoacuity steps, measured by parallactoscopometer for active (hatched columns) and passive (blank columns) movement ($n = 79$). Abscissa: Kinetoparallactic threshold values, mm (4.5 m in test distance). Ordinate: Respective numbers of test persons.

active dynamic parallactoscopy, could not be easily read from the statistical results. A comparably good value of 15 mm depth distance (Δ 60″ stereoacuity) was recordable from 25 percent of all probands. Active dynamic parallactoscopy of 45 mm (Δ 180″ stereoacuity) could still be sufficiently rated. Yet, when it comes to values worse than 45 mm, these would obviously be indicative of inhibited visual performance, so such values should be rated as pathophysiological. Good active dynamic parallactoscopy (30 mm depth distance, Δ 120″ stereoacuity) should, in any case, be required for professional and occupational activities where adequate assessment of three-dimensional situations is essential. The standard deviation is relatively high. Active dynamic parallactoscopy, therefore, may be assumed to be based on several separately variable optosensory factors that are independent of each other. Hence, excessive test values might possibly originate in an extreme situation from the summation of several equidirectional variants.

There seems to be good reason for the question of whether another degradation of depth distances might be in better compliance with the physiological aspects of dynamic parallactoscopy. Logarithmic degradation of optotype sizes was proposed by Schober (1976) for testing visual acuity, since such an approach seemed to promise better practice-related judgement of vision. This, however, would be hardly true for dynamic parallactoscopy and would simply make testing more difficult. That was the reason why linear graduation was chosen for earlier and more modern tests for measurement of the threshold of stereoscopy.

Total failure with regard to parallactoscopic stereoacuity is absolutely imaginable and comparable to stereo-amaurosis. However, a so-called central factor (Hofmann, 1925) of a kind that plays a considerable role in binocular stereoacuity, has not so far been described in the context of dynamic parallactoscopy, although it is quite certain that some sort of association by the central nervous system must be presupposed for transformation into a three-dimensional percept of the various velocities of contours moving in front of and behind a test object. Such involvement of a central factor might be expected only in individuals with severe cerebral lesions (Rennert, 1977).

Active dynamic parallactoscopy obviously constitutes a highly elementary performance of the visual cortex not bound to complicated associations like stereoscopic vision. Also, some factors which are important to binocular stereoscopic vision (e.g. binocular fusion, heterophoria, abnormalities of oculomotoricity, anisometropia, aniseikonia), seem to be unimportant to dynamic parallactoscopy, since this has proved to depend solely on monocular factors, above all, static visual acuity.

Passive dynamic parallactoscopy was determined with a fixed head and a stage width of 40 cm at a test object velocity of 0.5 m/s (see Section 3.2.3). The mean value of the detectable depth difference amounted to 2.9 cm throughout the routine examinations applied to the same probands who had been involved in testing for active dynamic parallactoscopy. The standard deviation was 1.6 cm. The frequencies of thresholds for all test persons are given in the bar chart of Fig. 9.

No significant difference was found to exist between active and passive dynamic parallactoscopy. The average threshold of stereoacuity amounted to 116″ for passive dynamic parallactoscopy.

4.2.2 Effects of age and static visual acuity

Kinetoparallactic vision is largely a combination of monocular optosensorial with oculomotorial requirements. Since both are associated with the central nervous system, effects of age are probable from the very outset, with the negative effects possibly being counteracted by experience and training. Yet, relatively low demands are made on sensoricity and motoricity by the parallactoscopometer. Only moderate active head and body movements are required. These can be determined by the probands themselves and are, thus, adjusted to individual capabilities. No extraordinary visual requirements are associated with the recognition of bars, since the diameter of the bars was 3.6 mm, which is enough for visual perception.

The partial correlation coefficients, after elimination of visual acuity and other remaining variables, were calculated for active as well as for passive dynamic parallactoscopy, with a view to ruling out, via age-dependent visual acuity, a direct influence of age. In this context, major differences were found to exist between the two types of movement. No age-related influence was recorded from active head and body movements, but a significant age-related influence was recorded from passive movements, the probable error being 5 percent.

The age dependence of passive dynamic parallactoscopy is of some relevance in real life, since there are numerous activities, in motorised road traffic and elsewhere, in which passive dynamic parallactoscopy is predominantly or exclusively required. In that respect, insufficiency may aggravate affinity between accidents, although the assumption can be made that decreased fitness might be offset by experience, training, attention, and caution, properties which have resulted in a general decline in accident rates in advanced age (see Section 4.1.2). Anyway, the man-vehicle-road complex (Lücking and Struppler, 1982) has been affected, through age-related involution, by several factors including dynamic parallactoscopy. For purposes of traffic safety medicine, attention should be given to age-related effects only in the higher decades of age (Gramberg-Danielsen, 1976). More reference is made to age-related effects on stereoscopic vision in Section 4.1.2.

It is in this context that some recognition is deserved of the findings regarding dynamic monocular visual acuity reported by Honegger, Schäfer and Jaeger (1969). Dynamic visual acuity values recorded by those authors from juvenile probands had been significantly better than those recorded from tests on persons of more advanced age. These findings were attributed to the delayed reactivity of people of higher age as well as to a general reduction of vision and, even more, to retarded and less accurate fixation in ocular pursuit, this also being of importance to dynamic parallactoscopy.

While lowered static visual acuity might imply reduced dynamic visual acuity, dynamic acuity cannot be automatically concluded from static acuity in an individual case, as was established in the comprehensive studies by Ludvigh and Miller (1958) and by Jaeger and Honegger (1964). It had to be found out whether static visual acuity was just loosely related to dynamic parallactoscopy or if there were inter-individual differences and to what extent impairment of general performance was to be expected as a consequence of reduced visual acuity.

While sizeable differences were found to exist between individuals across the group of 79 probands, static visual acuity was in direct proportionality to dynamic parallactoscopy. For example, the stereoacuity of probands with static vision between 0.4 and 0.6 amounted to about 50 percent of what were considered to be the normal values of dynamic parallactoscopy.

4.2.3 Effects of sex and occupational activity

A significant difference between both sexes was not recorded. As a matter of fact, such a difference could hardly be expected, since dynamic parallactoscopy is a sensory capability equal in either sex, just as are other categories of visual performance, say, visual acuity, scotopia, or limits to the field of vision. Almost all examiners have unsuccessfully tried to detect sex-related differences of stereoscopic vision.

Roughly 50 percent of all probands had higher educational backgrounds (university or technical school), so that two groups, skilled and unskilled, could be easily formed for comparison. Yet, no significant difference was established between the two groups in the course of evaluation.

Hence, educational background and occupational activity had no significant impact upon dynamic parallactoscopy, neither on dynamic stereoscopy (see Section 4.1.4). These findings applied equally to persons who were regularly involved in activities which called for good stereoscopic vision, such as workers in building construction, professional drivers, and craftsmen.

Dynamic parallactoscopy, just as visual acuity or dark adaptation, is a sensory quality basically possessed by any sighted individual – although with remarkable variations – with its level being unaffected by intelligence or education. Test results may, however, be affected by other individual properties and traits, such as capability of concentration, interest, and capacity of observation, as well as vigilance which may differ individually in persons, notwithstanding their occupations. Such traits and properties, however, are difficult to quantify and, consequently, cannot be reliably analysed.

4.2.4 Comparison between right and left eyes

The side of the eye for testing originally had been recorded for the purpose of completeness. Many examiners were surprised when statistical evaluation of eye-side comparison gave some strikingly unexpected results. With active movement, the parallactoscopy of the right eye was significantly better than that of the left (error probability being 5 percent). Differences were as great as 20 percent. However, no significant difference was recorded from passive movement.

This phenomenon can be primarily explained by monocular predominance. The optosensory impression on the right eye is predominant in about 85 percent of all human beings and is actually superior to that on the left eye. Left-eye predominance was recorded from about 10 percent of all the people examined, while 5 percent were ambidextrous, with no predominance of one eye being detectable. Percentual data are somewhat variable, depending on the methods used for examination, but right-eye predominance was overwhelming.

Such predominance is attributable to several factors, including much stronger involvement of the left cerebral hemisphere in all visual impulses. This principle of order has long been known and is also valid for hand- and leg-predominance. It is relatively labile but is, nevertheless, stable enough for unambiguous manifestation with high regularity in larger mass screening programmes. Diseases or blindfolding of the leading eye are much more troublesome to the affected individual than is the loss of the non-leading eye. The conclusion may be drawn from those interrelations that, in a comparison between both eyes in a monocular process requiring more than simply elementary vision, the leading eye would be capable of more effective vision than the non-leading eye. This is even more so in situations where adequate visual performance depends on associations with other cerebral regions such as the motor centres in the parietal brain. This is actually the case, if a proband who chooses his leading eye has to move both head and upper body for a better perception of a three-dimensional situation.

On the other hand, real object movements on a parallactoscopometer for testing passive dynamic parallactoscopy are possibly, by their very nature, too abstract and are without the involvement of any other cerebral regions, so that the predominance of one eye or a greater efficiency of the left cerebral hemisphere, will not be very effective. This appears to be in keeping with the observation that results of eye-predominance testing using Rosenbach's vision experiment, depend on a number of secondary factors including, for example, the hand in which the proband holds the pencil or turning of the proband's head.

4.2.5 Comparison between active and passive movement parallax

Almost identical performance levels were found to apply to threshold values of active and passive movement parallax or active and passive dynamic parallactoscopy (see Section 4.2.1), although they are two relatively independent and differently structured sensory functions, as may be seen from the differentiated effects of age and from a comparison of test results obtained from both right and left eyes. Yet, with all these structural differences, individual variations between these two versions of dynamic parallactoscopy are of minor importance.

This is an important conclusion, when it comes to practical handling of tests for dynamic parallactoscopy, as it shows that, even with a static test object, the effectiveness of dynamic parallactoscopy can be determined by means of active dynamic parallactoscopy, for example by using the common triple-bar apparatus, without any need for a relatively sophisticated parallactoscopometer.

Yet, the proband, in a seated position, should be given sufficient opportunity for unrestrained to-and-fro movement of head and upper body, not limited to two or three centimeters as had previously been the general practice of some authors (Cords, 1912; Perlia, 1911; Pfalz, 1907). In other words, no expensive apparatus, with motor drive, tachometer, and other gadgetry, is required to measure the individual efficiency of dynamic parallactoscopy.

5. Variations of test objects and testing methods

Almost all examiners, using a variety of different vision testing methods, have attempted to clear up the question of to what extent are test results affected by instruments or methodological modifications. All efforts made in that direction up to 1956, in the context of static stereoacuity, were collated by Linschoten. Römhild (1983) paid particular attention to instrumental modalities in connection with the triple-bar apparatus.

Many variations are also possible regarding test arrangements, test figures, and test apparatus for dynamic stereoscopic vision. These ought to be carefully analysed, the more so because there is no other hardware for verifying dynamic stereoacuity which has been shown to depend on two extremely sensitive components, stereoscopy and oculomotoricity. It is highly probable, therefore, that modifications of test conditions may be reflected in the results.

Also, several experimental series have been run with a view to identifying the best possible testing method for monocular dynamic stereoacuity. Ludvigh (1949) modified the circular diameters of object movements, optotype rpm, and luminance for three test persons.

The following experimental series illustrate the extent to which either type of dynamic stereoacuity can be affected by equipment, with special reference being made to the trends of such influences. Analyses of that kind are not only useful tools for critical appraisal of methods but are also of practical interest. They are likely to provide evidence that normal values are only of conditional relevance to workplace quality and road traffic or to any other field of life in which good dynamic stereoacuity is essential. They are also indicative of the wide-ranging variety of factors which have potential bearings on dynamic vision.

5.1 Dynamic stereoacuity

5.1.1 Various circular movements

Whenever dynamic stereoacuity is examined by means of prisms in synchronised rotation, it should be accepted that circular eye movements are involved and that a coordinative exercise of oculomotoricity is much more complicated than in the case of horizontal movements (Dieker and Honegger, 1968). For ocular pursuit of circular movements, the gaze is persistently forced to change directions with just as many corrective jumps. Hence, in response to the horizontal movement of optotypes, monocular dynamic visual acuity is about four times better than that in response to circular movement. Recordings of circular eye movements have also shown that ocular-pursuit moves could be made with low rpm values but gradually become detached from the test along with higher rpm values and extended pathways (Honegger, 1966). The ocular pursuit of an object in a circular movement, will be easier with angular velocity, rather than revolutions per minute, as the point of departure, if such a circular movement is of a larger radius. An increase in angular velocities with smaller circular radii will soon cause an increasing distortion of the ocular pursuit movement which ends up as an elliptical structure with an horizontal main axis. Ludvigh (1949), too, found that, with optotype movements in smaller circular orbits and by using weaker prisms to simulate rotation, visual performance decreased, in comparison to larger orbits, as long as angular velocity was the point of departure, i.e. the pathway travelled.

Rotating prisms of 4 prdpt tend to give a circular radius of 20 cm and a circumference of 125.7 cm for an observation distance of 5 m. The idea suggested itself that other prism thicknesses might as well be used to analyse dynamic stereoacuity, in order to take into account the factor sensomotor coordination in combination with stereoscopy. Tests were conducted, using 2, 4, and 8 prdpt with the circumferences of the circles, at an observation distance of 5 m, being 62.8, 125.7, and 251.3 cm, respectively. Angular velocity per second (°/s) could be calculated from rpm for each value, with due consideration being given to both the test distance and the circumference resulting from the deflection of prisms (Table 4).

The velocities, in m/s or in km/hr, reached at various speeds of revolution are of particular interest to occupational medicine and to road safety medicine in particular. The movements simulated by means of the rotational prismometer were little more than pedestrian or jogging speeds, as may be seen from the conversions in Table 5.

The results obtained from those comparative investigations and given in Figs. 10 and 11, support the following conclusions:

(a) Both two- and three-dimensional vision in pursuit of small circular movements were found to be better than the vision in pursuit of medium or large circular movements, with the same rpm (Fig. 10). The three curves in Fig. 10 differed significantly from each other, the error probability being 0.1 percent.

(b) Relations were almost inverted when the angular velocity was the point of departure (°/s): Circular movements with larger radii were then shown to be more easily controlled by the mechanisms of fixation and oculomotoricity and, consequently, enabled a more effective visual per-

Table 4. Conversion of rpm read from rotational prismometer to angular degrees per time second (°/s) for prisms 2, 4, and 8 prdpt in thickness.

Revolutions per minute (rpm)	Angular degrees per second (°/s)		
	2 prdpt $r = 10$ cm $u = 62.8$ cm	4 prdpt $r = 20$ cm $u = 125.7$ cm	8 prdpt $r = 40$ cm $u = 251.3$ cm
10	1.2	2.4	4.8
20	2.4	4.8	9.6
30	3.6	7.2	14.2
40	4.8	9.6	19.2
50	6.0	12.0	24.0
60	7.2	14.4	28.8
70	8.4	16.8	33.6
80	9.6	19.2	38.4
90	10.8	21.6	43.2
100	12.0	24.0	48.0
110	13.2	26.4	52.8
120	14.4	28.8	57.6
130	15.6	31.2	62.4
140	16.8	33.6	67.2

formance than circular movements with smaller radii, the travelling speed being unchanged (Fig. 11).

Prisms of 4 prdpt worked well on the binocular rotational prismometer for testing methods to determine both dynamic visual acuity and dynamic stereoscopy. The rpm values required on the apparatus were neither too high nor too low. Even more, eyes were not required to roam excessively.

One specific finding is that dynamic visual acuity in response to horizontal movement is better than that in the ocular pursuit of vertical or oblique movement (Ludvigh and Miller, 1958), but this cannot be automatically applied to stereoscopic vision, since the stereoscopic valency of vertical contours is much higher than that of horizontal contours. Also, the vertical

Table 5. Conversion of °/s on rotational prismometer to m/s or km/hr for 5 m observation distance.

m/s	°/s	km/hr
0.50	5.68	1.8
1.00	11.45	3.6
1.50	17.18	5.4
2.00	22.90	7.2
2.50	28.63	9.0
3.00	34.35	10.8
3.50	40.08	12.6
4.00	45.80	14.4

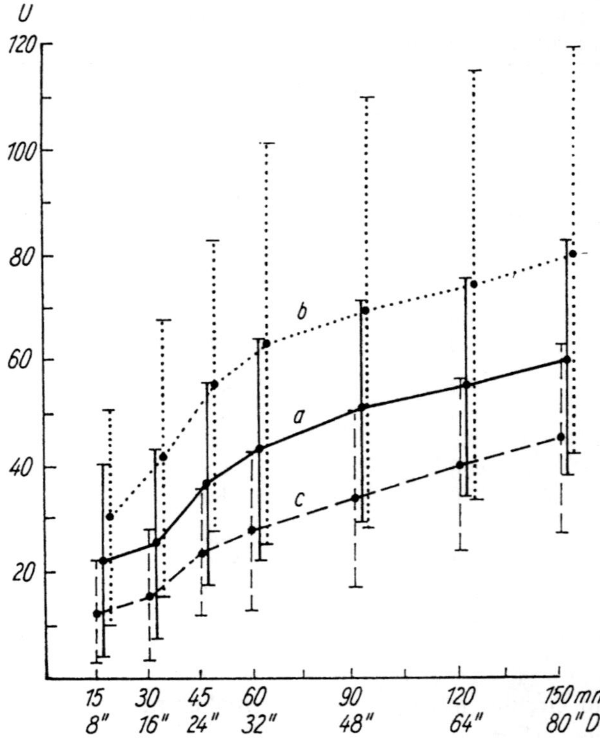

Fig. 10. Mean values and standard deviation of dynamic stereoacuity ($n = 10$) recorded from attachment to rotational prismometer of prism glasses of various strengths, depending on rpm. (*a*) Prism strength of 4 pdpt with equidirectional prism base of either side; (*b*) Prism strength of 2 pdpt on either side; (*c*) Prism strength of 8 pdpt on either side. Abscissa: Depth distance of bars (mm), and as angle of lateral disparity (*D*). Ordinate: Revolutions per minute.

structures of a vertically moved test object are perceived more intensively and for longer periods of time than the same structures of a target in horizontal movement. Experimental verification of these relations, however, is hardly possible, since reflector systems can be readily used to analyse monocular dynamic visual acuity in all directions of gaze, whereas rotary reflectors can just as well result in secondary non-stereoscopic factors of depth perception, so that it may be impossible to rate the quality of stereoscopy in isolation. For more reference to testing stereoacuity by means of polarisation techniques, see Section 2.2.2.

On the other hand, the suggestions made by Honegger and Schäfer (1968) on dynamic visual acuity with regard to vision with raised and lowered gaze, are also applicable to dynamic stereoacuity. Monocular dynamic visual acuity tends to deteriorate along with a raising of the gaze above 10 degrees or lowering below 20 degrees. In other words, visual quality tends to drop earlier and more intensively with a raising of the gaze, as compared to a

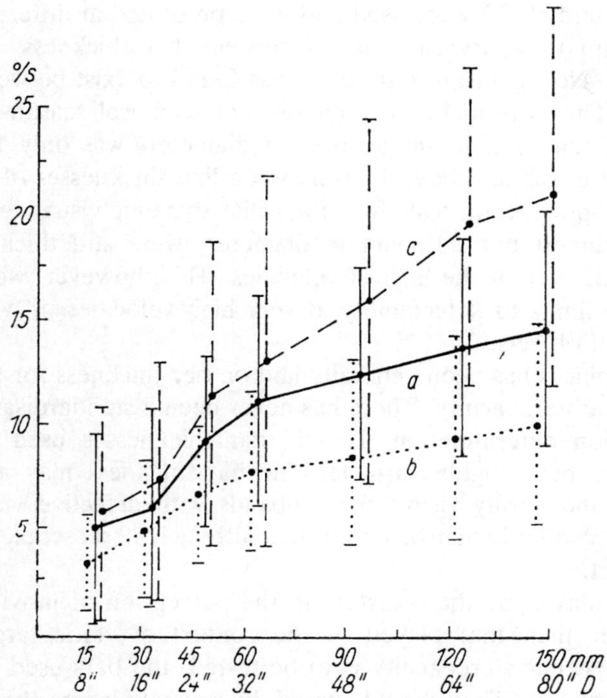

Fig. 11. Mean values and standard deviation of dynamic stereoacuity ($n = 10$) recorded from the attachment of prism glasses of various strengths to rotational prismometer, depending on the path (°/sec) travelled by the simulated image. Abscissa: Depth distance of bars (mm), and as angle of lateral disparity (*D*). Ordinate: Path in degrees per second. For *a*, *b* and *c*, see Fig. 10.

lowering. It is likely to reach its optimum at 5 degrees of lowering, which is the predominant gaze approximately taken in car driving and for a wide range of craft activities.

5.1.2 *Variations in bar thickness*

All tests so far applied to monocular dynamic visual acuity have shown that a straightforward correlation exists between the identifiability of optotypes and the quality of dynamic visual acuity. The larger and more easier detectable the optotype, the faster may be the movement with which the optotype can still be detected, although optotype detectability does eventually depend on bar or line thickness, when it comes to Landolt's rings or Pflüger's hooks. For dynamic visual acuity, Jaeger (1958) found that optotypes, 10′ in line thickness, could still be identified at an angular velocity of 50 °/s (circular movement), while those with 1′ line thickness were not identifiable at velocities above 10 °/s.

Bars with diameters of 1.8, 3.6, and 7.2 mm (giving angular apertures of

1′14″, 2′29″, and 4′57″) were used and were presented at different velocities in an attempt to verify correlations between bar thickness and dynamic stereoacuity. No significant difference was found to exist between the three test series. This is probably attributable, for technical reasons, to the fact that the ratio achievable among the bar diameters was only 1:2:4. However, the ratio was far above 1:10 between line thicknesses of the smallest and largest optotypes in tests for monocular dynamic visual acuity. Hence, even the thinnest bars, 1.8 mm in diameter, were still thick enough for identification, even at the highest velocities. This, however, would not rule out possible limits to detectability at very high velocities or with very thin bars or small objects.

Little emphasis has been generally laid on bar thickness for the measurement of static stereoacuity. There has never been a standardisation comparable to vision determination. Hence, bar thicknesses used by different authors have been highly variable. The bar thickness may appear to be inadequate and hardly visible for probands with defective vision, so that stereoacuity can no longer be confirmed, although stereoscopic vision might still be intact.

The role played by these factors in the perception of moving objects is even greater than that played in the context of static targets. Hence, whenever dynamic stereoacuity is to be tested, the bars used should be of sufficient thickness. They should exceed, by several factors, the visual acuity of the test person, lest the difficulty of perceiving moving details should not be additionally aggravated by the inadequate visibility of the test figure.

These relations are important in everyday life. Fast-moving small objects are inadequately localised in terms of three-dimensional perception, e.g. a brick dropping from a lorry in the traffic ahead and crushing the windscreen of a car or an insect flying into the face of a motorcyclist. Nevertheless, most events taking place in road traffic, in or out of movement, are identifiable, even under poor visibility conditions.

Comprehensive investigations were conducted by Aulhorn (1976) into static visual acuity in road safety medicine, e.g. distance of detectability, dependence on travelling speed, etc.

5.1.3 Variations in bar spacing

Many authors have noted static stereoacuity to deteriorate with a wider spacing of bars. Best (1949) and Römhild (1983) suggested an angle of vision of 17′ to be the optimum bar spacing, while about 30′ was considered to be optimum by Matsubayashi (1937). That difference between data has been attributable to the use of different types of measuring equipment. Under natural conditions of vision, stereoscopy tends to be outmatched by parallactoscopy and other empirical factors of three-dimensional perception, if the side-to-side spacing of bars is too wide. On the other hand, static stereoacuity is reduced if bars are too closely spaced. The problem of contour spacing is important to all methods of stereoacuity measurement, including those based on polarisers and anaglyphs.

Comparative investigations were conducted by means of the rotational prismometer (binocular), with midpoint bar spacings being 15, 30, 60, and 120 mm, with corresponding angles of vision of 10′, 20′, 41′, and 82′. Dependence of dynamic stereoacuity on midpoint bar spacings may be clearly seen from Fig. 12. Dynamic stereoscopy was favourably affected, along with high intensity, by wider midpoint bar spacings above a depth distance of 30 mm. Midpoint bar spacings, on the other hand, were less important in situations of smaller transverse disparations and lower velocities. At high velocity, a stereoscopic percept was more easily obtained from wider midpoint bar spacings than from narrower ones. Significant differences were found to exist between all test series, the probability of error being 0.1 percent. Those differences were primarily attributable to easier distinguishability and easier assessment of depth distances with wider bar spacings and under visual conditions of movement. The faster the movement, the more favourable would be a wider bar spacing which would enable easier detection of differences in bar positions. With smaller bar spacings, pictures of percepts of moving bars generally overlapped each other. Fast ocular pursuit movement, then, makes it impossible to dis-

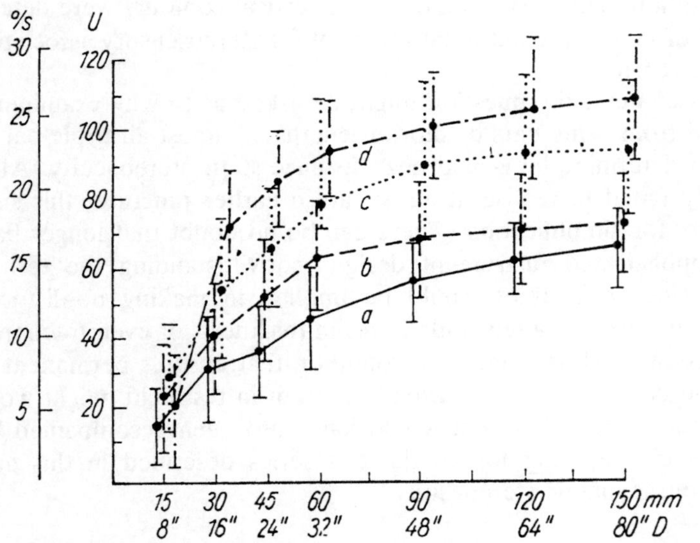

Fig. 12. Mean values and standard deviation of dynamic stereoacuity ($n = 10$) for different midpoint spacings of four bars. (*a*) 15 mm; (*b*) 30 mm; (*c*) 60 mm; (*d*) 120 mm. Abscissa: Depth distance of bars (mm), and as angle of lateral disparity (D). Ordinate: Revolutions per minute (right) and path in degrees per second.

tinguish between closely placed details of the same kind (e.g. the four bars of the test) and to compare them for three-dimensional visual perception. Assessment of a three-dimensional situation with fast movement is, in any case, easier if the contours involved are not too closely located to each other.

5.1.4 Variations in bar height

The question of how high bars should be for optimum test results has occasionally played a role, even with the triple-bar apparatus, and certainly under the assumption that a lower bar height would require a less comprehensive apparatus and, consequently, less designing and lower manufacturing costs. However, no interdependence was found to exist between bar height and depth acuity by Fruböse and Jaensch (1923). The same problem was experimentally treated, with the same result, by Best (1949) and Samsonowa (1936).

Shields can be attached to the upper and lower parts of the test platform so that the height of the test field on the rotational prismometer can be easily narrowed from 10 to 5, 2, or even 1 cm. Thus, an unambiguous result was obtained: dynamic stereoacuity was not reduced, even at a height of 1 cm. Even lower bar heights were not tested. These experimental findings were likely to support the conclusion that the length of the transverse disparate contours was unimportant to the visual cortex for three-dimensional localisation. The very condition that vertical contours were detectable in the field of vision, proved to be sufficient for stereosensory associations with the visual cortex.

In this context, the question might be asked as to why examiners always refrained from using bars of shorter lengths in almost all triple-bar arrangements to determine long- and near-distance static stereoacuity. All authors obviously failed to realise at all, or at an earlier juncture, this substantial possibility for simplification. There can be no doubt that longer bars entail more sophisticated instrument design, notwithstanding the test distance chosen, since difficulties would be implied in making no-distortion and no-curvature bars of a few millimetres in thickness, or even fractions of this, and of equal thickness and of a condition that ensures permanent straightness. The use of only 2 cm instead of 10 cm in test-field height would have yielded the same results but would have also been accompanied by fewer problems in preparing for all the test series described in this article for determining dynamic stereoacuity.

5.1.5 Depth distance of only two bars

The arrangements of the triple-bar and quadruple-bar tests have resulted from considerations at laboratory level and in terms of sensory physiology in which the practicability of the test procedures has played a somewhat important role, although in everyday life, situations are extremely rare in which such a kind of stereoscopy is required. For appraisal of stereoscopy, the triple-bar apparatus is based on six vertical limit contours. The four outermost contours have to be stereoscopically differentiated from the two that are centrally located. The quadruple-bar test is based on ten limit contours, including those of the side shield.

Presentation of only two bars would be closer to reality, with one of them placed forward and the other in a somewhat rearward position. Such situations are quite frequent in real life, e.g., a bar-shaped visual object, a branch or twig of a tree, or a length of wire which may have to be assessed for its three-dimensional arrangement relative to a similar visual object.

Many variants of the two-bar principle have been used in the past for static stereoscopy (Bishop, 1977; Howard, 1919; Matsubayashi, 1939; Verhoeff, 1933; Wagner, 1949). Hering and von Helmholtz have also used two bars in certain cases. All these authors had obviously been quite successful, but their approach was not adopted by their successors, although the two-bar procedure appeared to be superior to the triple-bar apparatus because of its clearer and more accurate physiological concept, and for being more elementary and easier to analyse. Yet, several contours are also presented by the modern stereoscopic polarisation tests. Six, for example, would be available from the polarisation-based Titmus ring test with its circles and circumference.

The applicability and suitability of two bars only had to be verified for testing of dynamic stereoscopy. Two bars, 3.6 mm in thickness and 3 cm in frontoparallel midpoint spacing without side shields, were used instead of four with side shields (Fig. 3d). One of the bars was pulled forward in steps of 15 mm. No horopter problems were encountered in the evaluation of this experimental arrangement, contrary to the triple-bar test where such problems clearly crop up in most cases (see Section 2.2.2). On balance, dynamic stereoacuity performance recorded from two bars was more significant (error probability 0.1 percent) than that recorded from the quadruple-bar test (Fig. 13). The reduction of vertical contours from 10 to four obviously had an enhancing rather than depressing effect on performance.

When it comes to monocular dynamic visual acuity, a great number of vertical contours no doubt facilitate assessment, primarily because of a stronger motivation for ocular pursuit movements. The optokinetic stimulus is certainly stronger, as it is not only supported by the detectability of one single structure but also by a great number of optokinetic details. A good example of this is the triggering of optokinetic nystagmus in response to a chessboard pattern. In the case of moving objects with depth distances, this optosensory situation will be further enriched by the extremely important time factor: little time will be left for the observer, during jumps of gaze (see Section 2.5), to visually scan all contours presented for different depths to

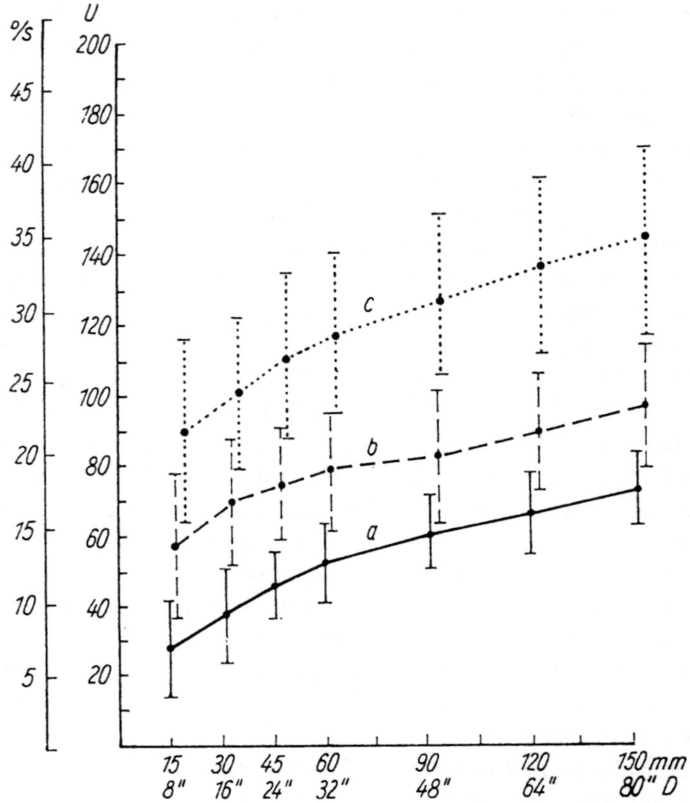

Fig. 13. Mean values and standard deviations of dynamic stereoacuity ($n = 10$) with the presentation of only two bars (*b*) and two plates (*c*) instead of four bars (*a*). Abscissa: Depth distance of bars (mm), and as angle of lateral disparity (*D*). Ordinate: Revolutions per minute (right) and path in degrees per second.

identify the limit contours that are relevant to final assessment. This necessary process of selection can be abandoned when only two bars are used.

However, the problem will be no more difficult to resolve with three bars in Hering's triple-bar apparatus (instead of four) in comparison to two bars, since the proband will have to focus attention only on one single (centrally positioned) bar. Hence, the high quality values obtained from the triple-bar apparatus are quite similar to those obtainable from two.

5.1.6 Depth distance of two surfaces

Assessment of the three-dimensional situation of two depth-different surfaces has proved to come even closer to the requirements of everyday life and occupational activity than the two-bar test arrangement, provided that the limit contours are not too far apart from each other. This is of particular relevance to road traffic. The surface limits of a vehicle must be compared and related to the position of another surface in many situations including pulling into a parking space or garage, overtaking, driving on tapered road sections, or convoy driving. Many similar examples are known from occupational medicine. However, the number of limit contours available for stereoscopic appraisal is further reduced to two when compared to a two-bar arrangement.

Two shields (black plates, 10 cm in width) were used instead of two bars. The side-to-side spacing between them was 3 cm. One of the shields was moved forward in steps of 15 mm. The person being tested had to tell which of the surfaces was further away. No additional contours of three-dimensional reference points were detectable on the right or left of the plates.

The test result is depicted in Fig. 13. The difference between four-bar and two-surface results was significant, the level of significance being 0.1 percent. A significant difference was also found to exist between results obtained from two bars, on the one hand, and those recorded from two plates, on the other, with the level of significance being 0.1 percent in favour of using two plates. Presentation of only two neighbouring limit lines of two plates actually reduces stereoscopic testing to the most elementary form. This approach has another advantage resulting from the absence of difficulties of detectability which otherwise could never be ruled out with three fast-moving bars and which would occur in this case only if contours were perceived as being out-of-focus. This may be the reason why the two-plate test figures gave values of dynamic visual acuity better than those recorded from any of the other test series. Hence, it is a major advantage that vision in everyday and occupational life is predominantly related to depth-distant moving surfaces. The precision of stereoscopy is surprisingly high at low travelling speeds. Results of the same quality were gained by using double triangles placed one upon the other (according to Cords, 1912), while, again, only two contours had to be rated, although disposed into two triangles (see Section 5.1.4 and Fig. 3f).

5.2 Dynamic parallactoscopy

5.2.1 Variations in bar thickness

Great importance must be attributed to the size or thickness of an optotype, or another moving object, if the latter is to be detected and properly identified. This has been borne out by investigations into monocular dynamic visual acuity (Jaeger and Honegger, 1964; Ludvigh and Miller, 1958; Schober, Munker and Grimm, 1967). However, it applies only conditionally to monocular dynamic parallactoscopy. The velocity of a test movement in a parallactoscopometer, nevertheless, will be unchanged after it was discovered that the quality of dynamic parallactoscopy was only affected to a minor extent within a wide range of medium velocities. A present unchanged velocity of 0.5 m/s (=6.3 °/s in 4.5 m distance) proved to be slow enough for the problem free detection of bars, 3.6 mm in thickness, even under dynamic visual conditions.

No significant test result differences were recorded from bar thicknesses of 1.8, 3.6, and 7.2 mm. However, in probands with visual acuity below 0.5, passive dynamic parallactoscopy was poorer in response to the use of very thin bars, as soon as the bar thickness fell below dynamic visual acuity (see Section 2.1).

5.2.2 Variations in bar spacing and bar height

The quality of stereoscopic vision of test figures with close and wide spacings among bars or contours, has been studied by numerous examiners of static stereoscopy (see Section 5.1.3). All authors found the quality of stereoscopic vision to deteriorate along with a wider spacings of bars, beginning with a visual angle of approximately 30 angular minutes (which would mean *ca.* 39 mm for a test distance of 4.5 m).

However, limitations in space were found to affect the verification of any relationships between dynamic parallactoscopy and bar spacing in a parallactoscopometer. Series of tests were run with bar spacings of 15, 30, and 60 mm (angles of vision of midpoint bar spacings with 4.5 m of test distance being 11′, 23′, and 46′).

Calculations of the significance of all midpoint spacings failed to reveal any noticeable difference. The adjustable lateral bar distances of the test configuration were obviously too small to produce any adverse effect of wider contour spacings upon the quality of dynamic parallactoscopy. Consequently, it was impossible to determine the bar spacing, critical for the parallactoscopometer, beyond which a deterioration of the test results would have to be expected. The midpoint bar spacings, adjustable on the parallactoscopometer, were obviously within an optimum range of values.

The effects of different bar heights in testing three-dimensional vision have been rarely studied in greater detail (see Section 5.1.4), probably because the extension or shortening of bars within a practicable range, would not produce palpable changes in test results. However, the question of what minimum length or size a visual object should have to provide optimum conditions for three-dimensional visual perception, is important in occupational medicine. No significant differences of dynamic parallactoscopy have been recorded from the triple-bar test, with visible bar heights being 12, 5, 2, and 1 cm.

These considerations, however, do not touch on the psychological aspects. Smaller visual targets would necessarily require greater attention from the proband and a greater effort will be needed for results of equal quality from very short bars. Such attention can be easily paid by the majority of probands for the period of a test, but a drop in performance is obsolutely possible in the context of protracted job exposure.

5.2.3 Depth distance of two and five bars

Two bars were found to be characterised by major advantages over three for dynamic parallactoscopy (see Section 5.1.5). No problem appeared to be involved in the preparation of such a test, since a high-accuracy setting of the spacings between bars was not necessary. The test problem is easy to explain and to understand, and is of an elementary nature in terms of sensory physiology because it is based on fewer contours (Fig. 3d).

The two-bar test was laid out in the same manner as the triple-bar test with regard to bar spacing, visible bar height, and bar thickness (see Section 3.2.2). Relative positions of the right or left bar in front or behind each other proved unimportant in test evaluation, although with frontoparallel movement, a rapprochement of bars was recorded in one case and a drifting apart, depending on the relative movement of the test object, in the other. Shifting the test towards the side of the rearmost bar would result in a rapprochement of both bars, which could be subjectively perceived with some certainty but was not measurable.

The following mean values and standard deviations of dynamic parallactoscopy (in angular seconds) were derived from the statistical data recorded from 10 probands: $136'' \pm 69''$ for two bars and $60'' \pm 25''$ for three bars. Test results obtained from two bars were worse than those recorded from three bars (error probability being 5 percent), in contrast to the values obtained from dynamic stereoacuity testing (see Section 5.1.5).

Five bars instead of three were rarely used in stereoscopy tests or were used for the sole purpose of accurately determining the threshold of three-dimensional perception. Examiners using five bars felt that appraisal might be facilitated by additional contours to flank the shiftable central bar (Mehlhose, 1975). Davidson (1935) required information from his probands as to which of the five differently placed bars was in the most forward or backward position.

There can be no doubt that a proband's attention is more intensively taxed if dynamic parallactoscopy is checked by more than three bars, since the individual tested would have to look at more contours and might be easily confused by a greater number of contours.

The central bar of the five (Fig. 3c) was shifted forward or backward for the testing proper ($n = 10$). Results obtained from this test arrangement were significantly worse than those recorded from the triple-bar test. Hence, when it comes to dynamic parallactoscopy, testing will become more difficult rather than easier when more than three bars are used.

5.2.4 Double triangular test

The double triangle (Fig. 3f) was first introduced by Cords (1912) with a view of determining the degree to which occupational fitness (degree of physical damage) was impaired by the loss of one eye. The bases of the two mirror-image superimposed equilateral triangles were not visible to the patient who was asked to push the cusp of the lower triangle precisely beneath the cuspidal point of the upper one (see Section 2.3.1). This apparatus, however, has never been developed beyond its experimental phase and, consequently, has neither been used for mass screening or for high-accuracy analysis.

The double triangle may be recommended for the measurement of dynamic parallactoscopy by means of a parallactoscopometer, since this test figure differs from bars, in that its detectability is widely independent of visual acuity. It is, therefore, particularly suitable for safe or reliable appraisal under conditions of movement and the objections made by Best (1949) are irrelevant to monocular movement parallax (see Section 2.3.1).

No significant differences were found to exist between the test results obtained from the double triangle, on the one hand, and those recorded from the triple-bar test, on the other. Mean values and standard deviations were 23 mm ± 14 mm ($n = 10$), with stereoacuity being 91″ ± 58″, when the double triangle was used, while the respective values with the triple-bar test were 20 mm ± 6 mm and 81″ ± 23″.

The preparation of a test for dynamic parallactoscopy, using a double triangle, proved to be much easier than that of a test configuration with three, four, or five bars. Hence, the more simple arrangement of the double triangle can be recommended to anyone intending to test dynamic parallactoscopy. Some interference factors likely to affect test results may, thus, be excluded, most of all from the influence of reduced visual acuity (see Sections 4.2.2 and 6.2.1), and the outcome will still be equivalent to that of the triple-bar apparatus.

5.2.5 Variations in image time and object speed

The effects of the length of image track, object speed, and image time cannot be checked separately from each other, since the three factors are interdependent. This is characterised by the formula $s = v \cdot t$ (s = image track, v = object speed, t = image time).

Dynamic stereoacuity was tested by means of a parallactoscopometer for image tracks of 10, 20, 40, and 80 cm. Object velocities were 0.12, 0.25, 0.5, and 1.0 m/s (Δ 1.6, 3.2, 6.3, and 12.7 °/s, under the assumption of a mean test distance). Resulting image periods were between 6.4 and 0.1 sec.

Involvement in the above-mentioned interdependence was not predictable for object velocity, although the speed of object movement had a major impact upon the threshold of dynamic visual acuity (see Section 2.1). The maximum movement adjustable on the parallactoscopometer amounted to 13 °/s (Δ 1 m/s Δ 3.6 km/hr). These were velocities at which any remarkable impairment of dynamic visual acuity could not be expected, the more so because the bars used were more easily detectable than optotypes would have been.

The above investigations ($n = 10$) showed, with an error probability of 5 percent, a significant dependence of stereoacuity on object velocity, in that stereoacuity worsened and the threshold of the stereoscopic vision increased in response to the increasing speed of the visual object (Fig. 14).

The detectability threshold of a given movement should be assumed, in the above context, as the minimum velocity and dynamic parallactoscopy would be impossible below that, with stereoscopic vision then being possible only on the basis of the time parallax (on the basis of successive comparisons of two positions at different junctures). The upper speed limit (with emphasis being laid on the angular velocity of relative movement between viewer and object rather than on real object speed) should be assumed to be the speed at which ocular pursuit movement is generally no longer possible or at which the decline in dynamic visual acuity would no longer permit the identification of a given object.

Dependence of image time on stereoacuity, by mathematical analysis (Fig. 15a), did not reveal any statistical correlation. However, it was clearly

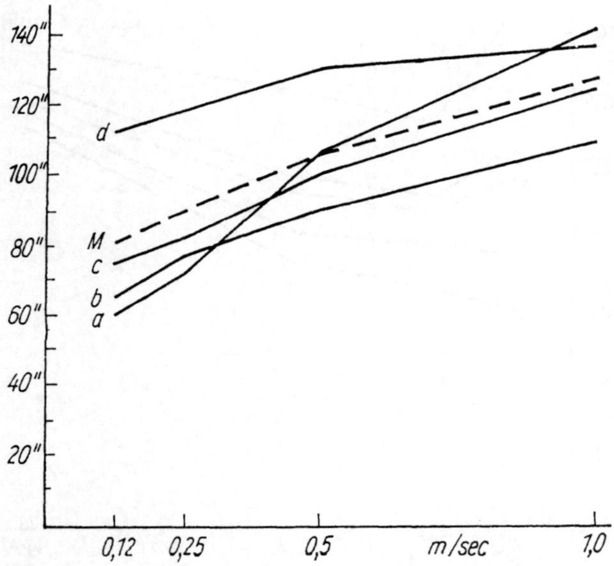

Fig. 14. Dependence of the threshold of movement parallactoscopy on object speed for various pathways of presentation ($n = 10$). (*a*) 100 mm; (*b*) 200 mm; (*c*) 400 mm; (*d*) 800 mm; *M* mean values of *a–d*. Abscissa: Object speed (m/s). Ordinate: Kinetoparallactic stereoacuity in angular seconds (").

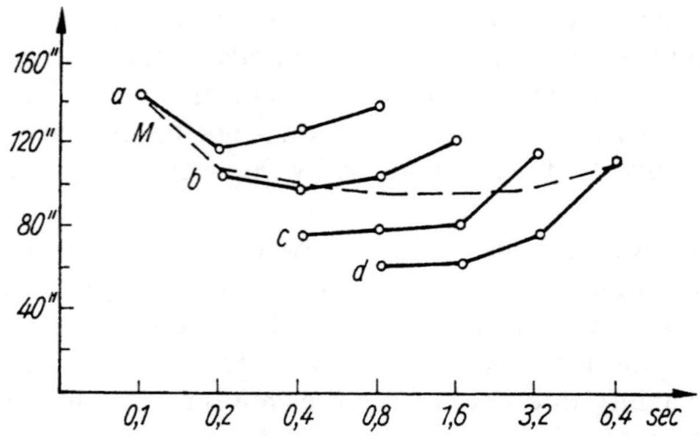

Fig. 15a. Dependence of threshold of movement parallactoscopy on time of presentation for testing with various lengths of presentation pathways ($n = 10$). (*a*) 100 mm; (*b*) 200 mm; (*c*) 400 mm; (*d*) 800 mm; *M* mean values of *a*–*d*. Abscissa: Presentation time in seconds. Ordinate: Kinetoparallactic stereoacuity in angular seconds (").

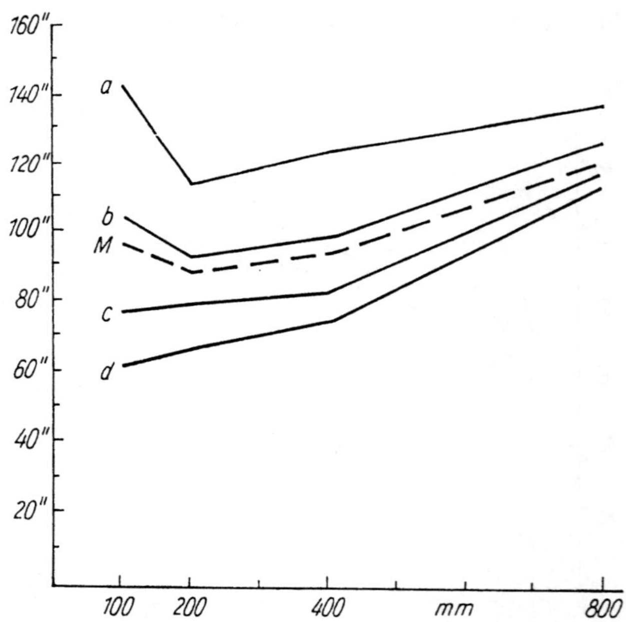

Fig. 15b. Dependence of kinetoparallactic stereoacuity on the presentation pathways for various velocities ($n = 10$). (*a*) 1 m/s; (*b*) 0.5 m/s; (*c*) 0.25 m/s; (*d*) 0.12 m/s; *M* mean values of *a*–*d*. Abscissa: Width of presentation pathway (mm). Ordinate: Kinetoparallactic stereoacuity in angular seconds (").

discernible that an optimum image time existed within the range of the test programme. Kinetoparallactic stereoscopic vision was at its highest efficiency for a viewing period of between 0.5 and 2 sec. An increasingly growing role, eventually leading to a decline in stereoacuity, was played by visual response time, when image periods dropped below 0.4 sec. A gradual decline in kinetoparallactic stereoacuity resulted from the growing use and increasing insufficiency of the optic memory when the image periods began to exceed 1.6 sec. Even longer image periods led to a level of predominance of the time parallax.

The length of an image track or observation path only had little impact on stereoacuity, along with optimum object speed, with such impact certainly being attributable only to the effect of speed on stereoacuity (Fig. 15b). Yet, the higher the object velocity, the longer the observation path pursued within optimum observation time will be, and the angle of observation will also be larger. This is a major advantage over stereoscopy. The basis of stereoscopy is virtually fixed by interocular distance and can be slightly enlarged only by means of expensive optical devices, whereas for dynamic parallactoscopy, the basis of movement parallax (viewing angle) can be freely selected. Hence, even at velocities around 6 m/s from a distance of 5 m, dynamic parallactoscopy is capable of detecting depth differences smaller than those identifiable by means of dynamic stereoscopy.

5.2.6 Variations in direction of movements

It has been one of the major advantages of dynamic parallactoscopy over dynamic stereoscopy, in addition to monocular vision, that disparations of oblique or vertical structures can also be utilised for three-dimensional orientation. In other words, a three-dimensional impression is visually generated on the basis of movement parallax by any kind of uniform movement. Since evidence has been presented on the dependence of the accuracy of ocular pursuit movements, not only on velocity but also on direction, parallactoscopic thresholds responding to passive movements (object movement with ocular pursuit movements) were compared with each other in different directions (horizontal, vertical, oblique) ($n = 10$).

Identical conditions were chosen for testing in all directions of movement. Bars were always vertically positioned in relation to the direction of movement. Automatic control for readjustment of performance levels enabled the maintenance of constant speed in both directions for vertical operation (see Section 3.2.1). A significant difference was found to exist between the horizontal direction of movement, on the one hand, and vertical or oblique directions, on the other. No difference at all was found to exist between vertical and oblique movements. The statistical data obtained from that investigation are given in Table 6.

Table 6. Results recorded from parallactoscopometer at different directions of movement ($n = 10$).

Direction of movement	Mean values	
	(mm)	(angular seconds)
Horizontal	16 ± 6	64″ ± 26″
Oblique (45°)	26 ± 12	103″ ± 46″
Vertical	24 ± 11	98″ ± 44″

Nevertheless, the results obtained from non-horizontal movements were only slightly poorer than those recorded from horizontal movements. That small difference might primarily be attributable to insufficient oculomotoricity which was a disadvantage, to say the least, to conditions of horizontal movement.

6. Dynamic stereoacuity in response to changes in perception conditions

The assumption that any reduction or impairment of visual perception might have adverse effects upon dynamic stereoacuity may well be justified. Precision and promptness of associations in the central nervous system might be affected, as well. It was, therefore, necessary to determine the extent of such an influence, together with relative important factors in order to gain more information about the structure of dynamic stereoscopic vision and its relevance to aspects of occupational medicine.

The aspects analysed in the series of tests that will be described in the following sections, are not merely of theoretical importance but can establish quantitative criteria. The visual handicaps reported were artificially induced, just as in the majority of similar laboratory experiments. The advantage of such an approach is implied by the fact that only one fresh interference factor or disorder has to be offset by a generally intact perceptive system, perhaps with the exploitation of so far unknown reserves, with lasting stress or pathogenesis of an asthenopic syndrome easily being avoidable. On the other hand, however, artificially induced conditions are always somehow strange and unusual. Individual probands may be assumed to cope with such conditions in different ways, and any kind of compensation will be individually variable. Also, all experimental series must proceed from a condition rated 'normal' in a preparatory ophthalmological examination without representing the maximum capability of the proband concerned.

A decisive role is played in everyday practice by adaptation of natural vision to any form of perceptive disorder. If a visual handicap develops during the course of life, some months or at least weeks have to be allowed for adaptation to the new status. This process is, to some extent, comparable to a process of training and exercise, as it will be initially characterised by a relatively drastic rise in performance (van Beuningen, 1949), lasting, however, only a few days or weeks from the onset of monocularity or some other visual defect. Further enhancement of performance will be at a slower rate but will still provide remarkable improvement. The latter is indispensable in road safety medicine, before such a monocular person can be accepted into motorised road traffic. The new visual defect will be gradually, but not completely, integrated with the associative systems of visual perception. That integration, however, is highly unsatisfactory in many cases.

A congenital visual defect or one acquired in early childhood, may have a severely adverse, often irreparable, impact upon the development and maturation of the visual sense. Synapses of the visual cortex and their connections to other cerebral regions, in such cases, cannot develop normally due to the absence of the necessary stimuli and may remain more or less rudimentary. On the other hand, there are some types of disorders resulting in development towards complete compensation for the given abnormality. Heterophoria is a good example in this context, its presence becoming a basis for the emergence of new control systems in the optosensory apparatus (Schober, 1976).

The objection appears to be somewhat justified that a visual handicap artificially induced to an otherwise ophthalmologically intact person is not really comparable to a defect of vision that had developed over a period of time. This certainly will be true in most cases. However, the experiment has an invaluable advantage, as it is based on more or less identical starter situations. In any case, the experimental investigations described below are closer to reality than many animal experiments. It goes without saying that only trends or directions of effects can thus be shown. Plenty of relative criteria for assessment are obtainable from experiments, and this is the specific value of them. Also, experiments have quite often surprisingly shown that the differences are not all that great between an artificially created situation and natural vision.

Additional importance should be attributed to experimentally induced disorders of dynamic stereoscopy, since comparable situations are not uncommon in reality. They may be caused by numerous different factors, e.g. dimmed lighting, glare, obstruction of vision by fog or rain-wetted or dirty windscreens, pseudoheterophoria due to decentered eye glasses, or artificial refraction abnormality because of wrong eye glass values. Such situations, however, have rarely been recorded in the realms of occupational activity due to stringent industrial safety and job fitness regulations. These are just some of the transient interference factors through which dynamic stereoscopy, sufficient for normal every-day life, might prove to be insufficient.

Binocular functions are of relatively recent origin in terms of phylogenesis. That is why the effects of noxae on dynamic stereoscopy are much greater than on light or colour perception and on visual acuity. These are elementary factors of the very early origin in phylogenesis.

The spectrum of possible effects will be analysed below together with the effectiveness of each of the factors involved.

6.1 Dynamic stereoacuity

6.1.1 Bilateral impairment of visual acuity

Substantial deviations have been recorded from different statistical records regarding incidence of bilaterally impaired visual acuity in a given population. The age groups of probands have been of crucial importance. In Central Europe defective vision below 0.2 has been recorded from 0.1

percent of probands aged 45 years, 0.2 percent aged 50, and 5 percent of all people aged 60 years (R. Sachsenweger, 1972).

Linschoten (1956) found the effect of visual acuity on static stereoacuity to be considerable. An almost linear relationship was found by van Beuningen (1948), Haberkorn (1965), and Levy and Glick (1974), to exist between impaired visual acuity and reduced stereoscopic vision. Stereoscopic vision was believed to be disrupted in response to a visual acuity of 0.1 (Colenbrander, 1948). Heinsius (1944) verified good static stereoacuity only up to 6/6 vision of both eyes. Lorenz (1943) denied the existence of a somewhat closer correlation between visual acuity and depth acuity for probands with average visual acuity values. Schneider (1981) suggested that bilateral aphakia was accompanied by a decline in stereoacuity along with a decrease in visual acuity of the poorer eye. However, most of these data were based on measurements, using methods which prevented any generation of stereoscopy because of too few test details. Lang (1982) proposed rudimentary stereoscopy to continue, even in parallel to severe weakness of vision, provided that the visual test objects were large enough.

For the following investigations, visual acuity of both eyes was artificially reduced to $V = 0.6$, 0.4, 0.25, and 0.1 by means of Bangerter opaque screens. Their effectiveness was highly variable on account of technical irregularities. All screens were, therefore, checked for vision-reducing effectiveness, prior to application. Bar width was 7.2 mm in the quadruple-bar tests of this series to make adequate allowance for reduced visual acuity.

Results obtained from tests of dynamic stereoacuity in 13 normally sighted probands are given in Fig. 16. Dynamic stereoacuity may be seen to approximately drop to the extent to which visual acuity is reduced in both eyes, though at a much lower rate. A significant difference was shown to exist among curves for bilateral reduction of vision to $V = 0.6$, $V = 0.4$, and $V = 0.25$. When vision was reduced to $V = 0.1$, only eight in 13 probands had a depth percept of 150 mm and only four had one of 60 mm. Probands with excellent static stereoacuity generally exhibited above-average dynamic stereoscopy, even with screens on their eyes.

The fact that dynamic stereoacuity was reduced only to a minor extent after artificial bilateral reduction of vision was remarkable. Yet, the bars of the test figure were easily visible, even for probands with poor visual acuity. Stereoacuity would have declined much more drastically along with reduced vision, had thinner bars been used.

The relatively minor impairment of dynamic stereoacuity in response to a bilateral reduction of vision was particularly conspicuous by the following comparison: reduction in visual acuity from 1.0 to 0.1, that is from 100 to 10 percent, was followed by 50 percent drop in dynamic stereoacuity. Stereoacuity deteriorated by only about a quarter of normal performance, when vision was reduced to 0.25. On the other hand, there were some probands in whom dynamic stereoacuity underwent almost total collapse due to a very slight reduction of vision.

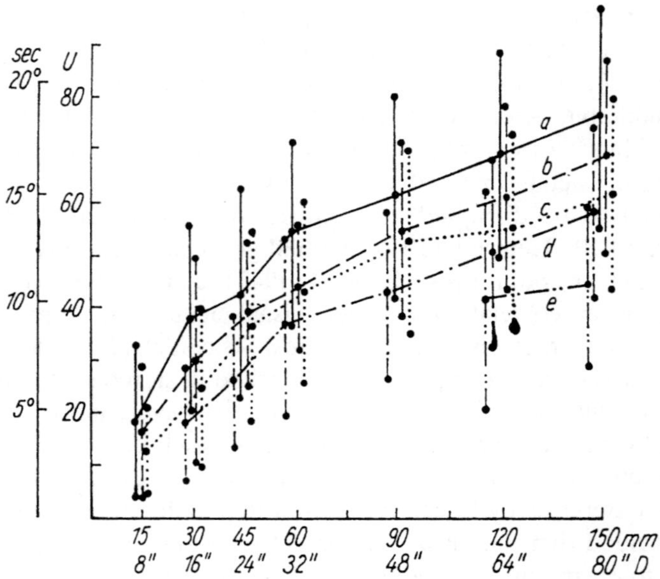

Fig. 16. Mean values and standard deviation of dynamic stereoacuity ($n = 13$) in response to an artificial reduction of the visual acuity of both eyes, using screens. (*a*) Without screens; (*b*) Reduction of visual acuity to 0.6; (*c*) 0.4; (*d*) 0.25; (*e*) 0.1. Abscissa: Depth distance of bars (mm), and as angle of lateral disparity (*D*). Ordinate: Revolutions per minute (right) and path in degrees per second.

Similar findings were reported by Helveston and von Noorden (1967), Lang (1982) and Roggenkämper (1983) who agreed that stereoacuity, with regard to unmoved objects, could be surprisingly good, even with reduced vision. With easily detectable test objects, only relaxed relationships obviously exist between visual acuity and depth acuity, since visual acuity is based on the retinal resolution power of the eye, whereas stereoscopy is based on a functional system within the visual cortex usually activated by perception of the entire test figure.

Protracted weakness of vision in childhood has quite often led to stereoamblyopia, with stereoscopic vision then being clearly poorer than in response to an artificial reduction of vision. However, when it comes to individuals in whom visual acuity had recently deteriorated, the effect of pathological alterations is identical to that caused by artificial impairment.

There are plenty of practical examples of the artificial bilateral reduction of visual acuity, especially in road traffic, i.e., due to scratched or soiled goggles of motorcyclists, opalescence and interfering reflections due to rainfall, smudged or iced-up windscreens of motorcars, etc. Myopia and hyperopia up to ±2.0 dpt as well as astigmatism up to cyl ±6.0 were artificially induced in 10 probands in four series of tests. In these investigations, dynamic stereoacuity was found to be adversely affected in parallel with a reduction of visual acuity, owing to refractive abnormality.

6.1.2 Unilateral impairment of visual acuity

Unilateral impairment of vision has been proved to occur with much higher frequency than bilateral reduction of visual acuity, even without approximate data on its incidence in the general population. The possible guess for Central Europe is about 20 percent of all people with vision below 0.3 in one eye and 10 percent with vision poorer than 0.1, people in advanced age included. Much lower figures, however, would result from reference to the records of physical inspection for military service and school entry examinations. Many affected individuals are not even aware of their insufficiency until they decide to go for a job where intact bilateral vision is necessary. Strabism and strabismic amblyopia may be causative factors of major importance.

Only a few communications have so far been made available on the unilateral reduction of visual acuity and its bearings on static stereoscopy, with most of them referring to small groups of patients. Jofe (1937) found static stereoacuity to depend on the difference that existed for visual acuity between the two eyes of a proband, provided normal vision of one eye and normal stereoacuity as long as visual acuity of the poorer eye has not dropped below 0.4. However, under static conditions, Best (1949) found some parallelism between a reduction of stereoacuity and the vision of the poorer eye. Colenbrander (1948) suggested that static stereoacuity was no longer measurable if the vision of one eye had dropped to 0.1. Heinsius (1964) found static stereoacuity reduced, even in response to monocular impairment of visual acuity below 1.

The methodological approach chosen for the following test series with an artificial unilateral reduction of vision, was identical to that taken for binocular impairment of vision. The left eye was kept at normal vision.

Unilateral artificial impairment of vision conspicuously affected dynamic stereoacuity more severely than bilteral impairment. This may be seen from the test results in Fig. 17. Average dynamic stereoacuity for a bilateral and unilateral reduction of vision to 0.6, 0.4, and 0.25 is depicted as a relevant example in Fig. 18. The difference is significant. Differences between both in response to lower velocities are more strongly pronounced than the differences with higher velocities.

Studies into optosensory performance under conditions of unilaterally reduced visual acuity are much more important than studies into conditions of bilateral impairment for several reasons: the number of affected people is much higher. The view is widespread that a unilateral reduction of vision would not entail palpable disadvantages in the general performance of the optic sense organ. The impact of the unilateral reduction of visual acuity on dynamic stereoacuity is significantly worse than that of a bilateral reduction. Optimum functionality of binocularity obviously depends on adequate information from both eyes which must be the same in terms of quality and

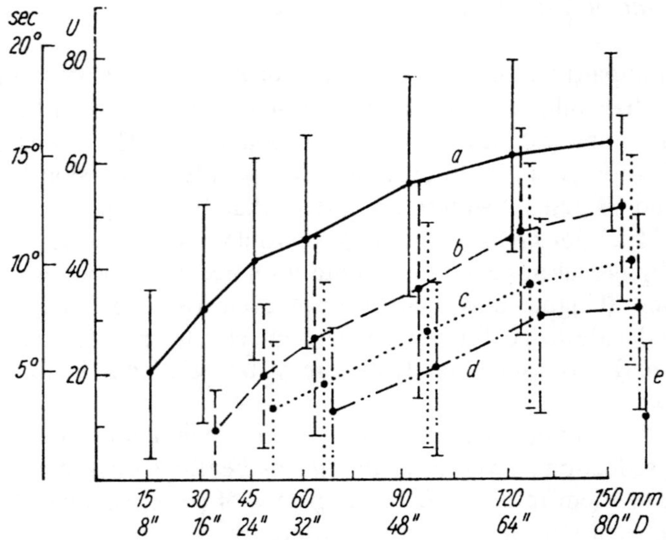

Fig. 17. Mean values and standard deviation of dynamic stereoacuity ($n = 10$), following an artificial monocular reduction of the vision of the right eye, using screens. (*a*) Without screens; (*b*) Vision of 0.6; (*c*) 0.4; (*d*) 0.25; (*e*) 0.1. Abscissa: Depth distance of bars (mm), and as angle of lateral disparity (*D*). Ordinate: Revolutions per minute (right) and path in degrees per second.

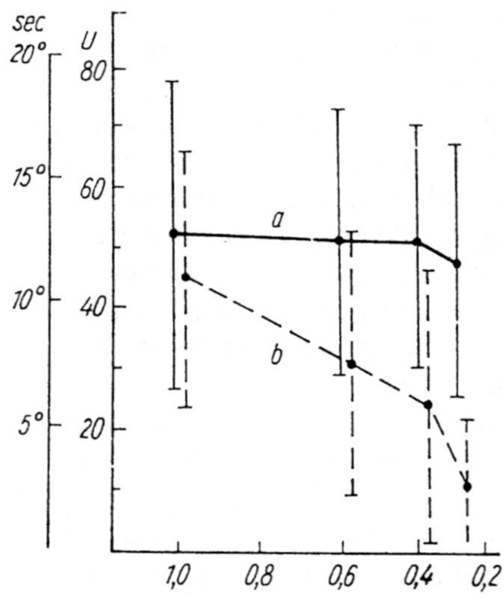

Fig. 18. Mean values and standard deviation of dynamic stereoacuity ($n = 10$), following bilateral (*a*) and unilateral (*b*) reduction of visual acuity by means of screens. Abscissa: Visual acuity in decimal values. Ordinate: Revolutions per minute (right) and path in degrees per second.

quantity. Inadequate stimuli can be more easily and more effectively compensated under static conditions. However, insufficiency will become obvious and will be seriously felt, if the factor of interference is added, as would be the case with watching moving objects.

In this context, a decisive role is played by binocular fusion, as had been established in earlier investigations (M. Sachsenweger, 1979). The weakening of fusion intensity as a result of the unilateral reduction of vision was much more severe than that caused by bilateral impairment. The same results were reported by Aust (1978), following his investigations on the width of fusion in the wake of binocular and monocular reduction of visual acuity. The quality of stereoscopic vision is substantively determined by the poorer eye, even after an extended period of monocular impairment of visual acuity (Best, 1949). The fact that dynamic stereoacuity is more adversely affected by monocular vision impairment than by binocular reduction, may be of relevance to fitness for certain occupational activities.

6.1.3 Conditions of scotopic vision

Visual capability under scotopic conditions is very important: Roughly 25 percent of all road traffic accidents were found to have occurred at dawn or dusk, despite a lower traffic density. One-third of all accidents, and even more, falling accidents, were found to occur under artificial lighting. The lowest accident rates in many statistical records are in June, the month with the longest daylight periods, and the highest are recorded in January, although additional factors might be involved (Aulhorn, 1976; Bockelmann, 1982).

The steadily growing motorisation and more effective utilisation of all means of road transport have necessarily increased night travelling in recent years. At present, the severity of road accidents and the overnight casualty rate are twice as high as those in daytime, if allowance is made for traffic density. That is the reason why more attention has been paid recently to analyses of visibility conditions for night travelling. The difficulties implied in scotopic vision are characterised by extraordinary dynamics, since visibility for road driving is subject to constant change (Kronesser, 1981). Job fitness regulations for drivers in most countries are quite tough, and for good reasons, with regard to reduced scotopic and night vision.

The question for the intensity by which dynamic stereoacuity is affected may be of additional interest with reduced luminance in road traffic. Light cones of vehicular headlights are absolutely straight in orientation, while targets for three-dimensional perception are usually lateral from the cone, e.g., in curve driving, pulling into parking spaces or pulling back. The luminance values of properly illuminated roads at night, and of roads with bright pavement, are rarely below something between 3 and $0.3\,cd/m^2$ ($1\,cd/m^2 = 3.1416\,asb$). The luminance values in light cones of vehicles on country roads at night are between 1 and 0.1 cd/m^2 and tend to go down to something between 0.1 and 0.01 cd/m^2 at a distance of 50 m from the headlight. Hence, apart from the road section just ahead of the travelling car, darkness driving on a country road will impose conditions of mesopic vision on the driver (Aulhorn, 1976) ranging from about 0.3 to 0.003 cd/m^2.

Without supporting artificial lighting, luminance values are between 0.1 and 0.03 cd/m^2 in full moonlight, 0.01–0.003 cd/m^2 under new moon conditions, and 0.003–0.0003 cd/m^2 with starlit skies. Luminance values of 0.003 cd/m^2 tend to cause an onset of the Purkinje effect (central scotoma with loss of colour vision) and Kohlrausch's break in the adaptation curve.

Apart from transport-related and other special occupations, however, dynamic stereoacuity under conditions of scotopic vision is probably not too important, as most occupational activities are carried out under sufficient to optimum lighting conditions. Yet, in private life, dynamic vision under twilight conditions may be more important, since the individual is quite often required to move in relative darkness.

Little attention has so far been given to the quality of stereoacuity under conditions of scotopic vision. Studies in the past had been remarkably scarce and inadequate to poor with regard to the luminance values used. Results so far communicated have been variable. Heinsius (1964) explained those shortcomings by reference to technical problems.

Systematic studies into static stereoacuity under conditions of reduced luminance (R. Sachsenweger, 1954) showed that stereoscopic values dropped drastically as of 1 asb, while larger variations were recorded from low luminance levels. Most of that interindividual scatter was based on the scatter in adaptation curves of people with normal vision which differed by a ratio of 1:5 (Piper, 1951). Fruböse and Jaensch (1923) suggested that stereoacuity in average daylight was inferior to that in very bright artificial lighting. Three-dimensional vision in twilight with monocular viewing was compared by Glees (1949) to three-dimensional vision in twilight with stereoscopy. The results obtained from stereoscopic vision were 18 times better, suggesting considerable importance of stereoscopy to three-dimensional orientation under conditions of scotopic vision. Stereoscopic vision, according to Schumann (1959), disappeared if luminance dropped below 1 lux. Monje (1969) found static stereoacuity to be reduced, even in conditions in which unambiguous foveal vision was still possible.

Static monocular visual acuity has quite often been tested in the past under conditions of reduced lighting and has proved to be almost normal with a surrounding field luminance of between 100 and 10 asb (vision being somewhat above 1). It was found to drop to about 0.7, with 1 asb (the beginning of scotopic vision), and to about 0.3 in response to 0.1 asb. The subsequent decline would be very steep (Aulhorn, 1976).

Studies into monocular dynamic visual acuity, especially in the context of high luminance values, were conducted by Honegger and Alexandridis

(1970). A Tübingen-type projection perimeter with rotating prism was used in these tests. The higher the adaptive luminance (background brightness), the less strongly pronounced was the decline in visual acuity for moving objects along with higher angular velocities of optotypes.

Combined testing of vision, as well as perception of contrast and glare, would be very important in the proper assessment of driving capabilities in the mesopic context (Schmidt, 1976). Attempts were made to establish whether or not dynamic stereoacuity ought to be included in such combined test arrangements, at least in selective cases. The luminance levels of a test field by means of a connected transformer were reduced in a stepwise manner to 3.19, 0.319, and 0.032 cd/m^2. The test room was totally blacked out and was then illuminated only by the test surface. Testing was started with a luminance of 31.9 cd/m^2, a value at which optimal vision testing was only conditionally possible, according to Schober (1976). The examiners then proceeded to lower the luminance levels. Each of the persons being tested was given about 10 min for adaptation to changing visual conditions.

The result of that test programme is depicted in Fig. 19 and is compared to the outcome of a mass screening with a luminance of 620 cd/m^2. Considerable inter-individual variations were recorded in response to low luminance. Dynamic stereoacuity was found to gradually become insufficient in response to the decrease in luminance, although more slowly than originally expected. Nevertheless, values were no longer measurable from

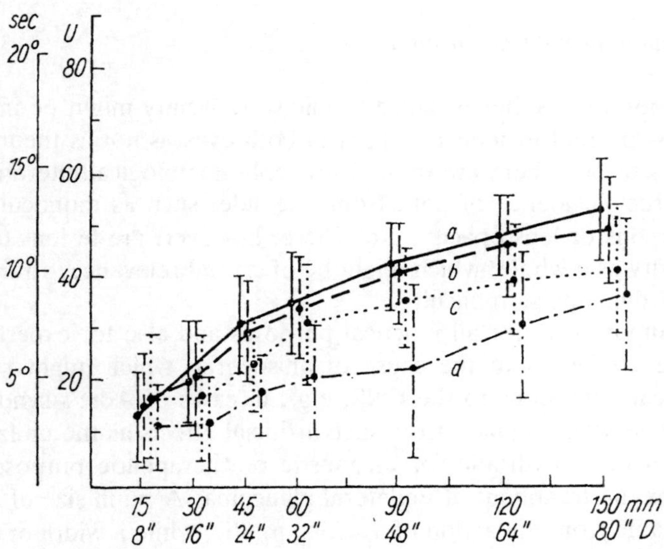

Fig. 19. Dynamic stereoacuity with standard deviation ($n = 10$) for reduced luminance levels. (*a*) 60 cd/m^2; (*b*) 31.9 cd/m^2; (*c*) 3.2 cd/m^2; (*d*) 0.3 cd/m^2. Abscissa: Depth distance of bars (mm), and as angle of lateral disparity (*D*) in angular seconds ("). Ordinate: Revolutions per minute (right) and path in degrees per second.

any of the test persons when luminance had dropped to 0.03 cd/m^2. Very general data of dynamic stereoscopy began to be recorded from about 0.15 cd/m^2. The differences between the curves were significant, with the probability of error being between 0.1 and 5 percent. Immediate sensory causes included unreliable fixation as well as decelerated and deviating ocular movements in visual pursuit of moving objects under twilight conditions. This had been established by Honegger and Schäfer (1964) in their investigations into monocular dynamic visual acuity. Ocular pursuit and corrective movements have been shown to be severely impaired and inhibited under conditions of scotopia. The fixation reflex of the foveola was found to be reduced, even if the intensity of the stimuli was still sufficient under static conditions. Also, the time required for binocular fusion was found to continuously increase along with declining luminance, according to Piper (1951). Additional important effects were also found, including a reduction of visual acuity, depending on luminance, the need for adaptation to the dark with its inevitable darkness mydriasis, incipient central twilight scotoma, and nocturnal myopia. The fatigue factor is no less important due to the existence of profoundly psychic correlations between scotopic vision and fatigue.

There are quite a number of situations of scotopia in which the importance of empirical, secondary factors of depth perception of moving objects (movement parallax, dimensions, perspective, overlapping of contours, etc.) can be even greater than in stereoscopy.

6.1.4 Unilateral light absorption

The question of whether or not dynamic stereoacuity might be impaired by the latero-different incidence of light to both eyes, is not as theoretical as it first seems to be. There are quite a few ophthalmological alterations which may obstruct incidence of light from one side, such as monocular corneal scars, vitreous or lens opacity, etc. These, however, are lesions to suppress visual acuity as a whole, which might be of crucial relevance, after all, to the quality of dynamic stereoacuity.

More importance, for all practical purposes and also for expert opinions, should be attributed to the cause of anisocoria, which might result from pathological alterations to the CNS, e.g., in cases of Adie's syndrome, but might just as well originate from such artificial effects as the unilateral drop application of a mydriatic for diagnostic or therapeutic purposes or of a mioctic for the treatment of unilateral glaucoma. A pupil size of 2 mm may be recordable from the action of a strong miotic, while a width of 8 mm may result from a strong mydriatic. Light incidence to a pupil of 8 mm in diameter is more than 15 times higher than in a pupil of 2 mm.

The effect of monocular light absorption glasses has been studied by several authors in the past and has some surprising insights. Improvement in static stereoacuity by up to 45 percent was found by Schaefer and Ebner (1948). Their findings were further increased to 75 percent when grey glasses were used. Haberkorn (1965), using unilateral light absorption of something between 80 and 90 percent, recorded an improvement in static stereoacuity by something between 12 and 36 percent. Similar investigations were reported by Monje (1947), Münster (1942), and Verhoeff (1933). No reports have so far been produced on observations to the contrary.

A differentiated incidence of light was achieved by the application of a (Heliosal) glass for 75 percent light absorption to the right eye. Dynamic stereoacuity appeared to be slightly enhanced, though the difference was not significant. Eight in 10 persons tested felt light absorption glasses to be pleasant or vision-supporting.

It has not been easy to find an explanation for such an enhancement, although it had been a subjectively perceived phenomenon. There might be something similar to the Pulfrich phenomenon where more impressive stereoscopic perception was found to arise from unilateral application of a light absorption glass due to different conduction velocities along the two visual pathways, on account of the action of unequal brightness.

Yet, the assumption, seems to be more strongly supported that the competition between the two eyes might have been activated by latero-different brightness perception, particularly as that competition, according to Hamburger (1952), is not only a substantial prerequisite for binocular vision but is also essential to its quality. The action of unequal stimulation energies on the two retinae, optokinetic adjustment movements, or different impulse patterns in the pathways of the two eyes, were considered by Haberkorn (1967) to be causes of improved depth acuity.

6.1.5 Anisometropia

If consideration is given to low anisometropies (i.e. latero-different ametropies), there will be only a few people without any anisometropia. There are also many people with relative emmetropia, i.e. with unequal refractivity of the refractive media of the eye, which would give emmetropia again, particularly as all refractive media of the eye vary strongly. Many of them are absolutely independent and separate. Anyway, abnormal refraction of one refractive medium has quite frequently been offset by the abnormality of another. Anisometropia, measurable by skiascopy, was found to be recordable in 50 to 80 percent of all human beings, depending on the criteria and age groups. Variations in bulbar length were found to be the most common causes. No correlations were found to exist between handiness and anisometropia.

Anisometropia patients may differ from each other in their vision. Severe anisometropia may prevent binocular vision and may, quite often, even provide a basis for unilateral amblyopia.

The quality of static stereoacuity, in cases of slight and medium anisometropia, generally depends on the visual acuity of the poorer eye (Best, 1949; von Beuningen, 1948; R. Sachsenweger, 1954). Impairment of vision due to anisometropia, is primarily attributable to a difference between the two sides in an accommodation effort, particularly as the capability of laterally differentiated accommodation is limited. Differentiated prismatic deflection after laterodifferent eyeglass correction may be another factor leading to anisophoria. Anisophoria is particularly felt with upward or downward gazes, as in reading, since these gaze directions have only a narrow width of fusion. Aniseikonia is another problem, next to anisophoria, which is usually tolerated, depending on constitution and age.

Against the background of the high incidence of anisometropia among the general population, it was of some interest to find out to what extent dynamic stereoacuity was affected by it. Anisometropia was simulated by the experimental induction of myopia or hyperopia, using +1, +2, +3, −1, −2, and −3.0 dpt. In all cases, glasses were placed in front of the right eye.

The results obtained from 10 persons tested are depicted in Figs. 20 and 21. A significant difference of +1 or −1 dpt was found to exist between responses by persons tested without artificial anisometropia, on the one hand, and those with anisometropia, on the other. No significant difference was recorded from a comparison of results obtained from artificial myopic

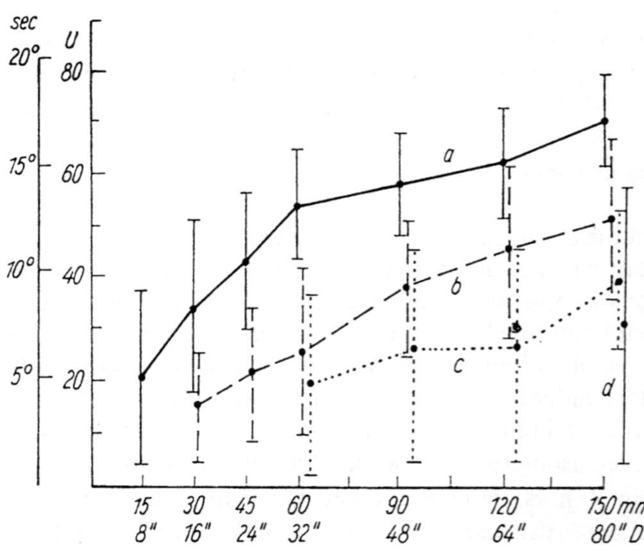

Fig. 20. Dynamic visual acuity with standard deviation ($n = 10$) in the case of artificially induced hyperopic abisometropia (left eye remaining emmetropic). (*a*) Without anisometropia; (*b*) With −1.0 dpt in front of right eye; (*c*) −2.0 dpt; (*d*) −3.0 dpt. Abscissa: Depth distance of bars (mm), and as angle of lateral disparity (*D*). Ordinate: Revolutions per minute (right) and path in degrees per second.

anisometropia, using +1.0 dpt, on the one hand, and those from hyperopic anisometropia, using −1.0 dpt, on the other. Too few couples were available for the statistical significant calculation of myopic and hyperopic anisometropia by ±2.0 dpt, since, even with substantive lateral disparity, measurable dynamic stereoacuity was recordable from only five in ten of the persons tested with artificial anisometropia of such a magnitude. Hence, even the graph remains incomplete.

These studies are likely to provide evidence for the severe impairment of dynamic stereoacuity due to anisometropia, with the loss of actual visual acuity occurring independently. For example, in two of the 10 probands, dynamic depth acuity collapsed, even in response to a one-sided application of −1 dpt, although vision as such was negligibly reduced and, theoretically, compensation should have been possible by increased accommodation.

Static stereoacuity may be affected by differences in refractivity as small as 0.5 dpt, according to van Beuningen (1948) and R. Sachsenweger (1954). Best (1949) found that even an experimental anisometropia of 2 dpt might support a trend towards the abandonment of stereoacuity in favour of easy monocular vision, i.e. transition to monocular suppression. Yet, measurable stereoacuity of up to 6 dpt was exhibited by cases of congenital anisometropia unless strabism had developed.

It seems quite obvious that especially dynamic stereoacuity is considerably

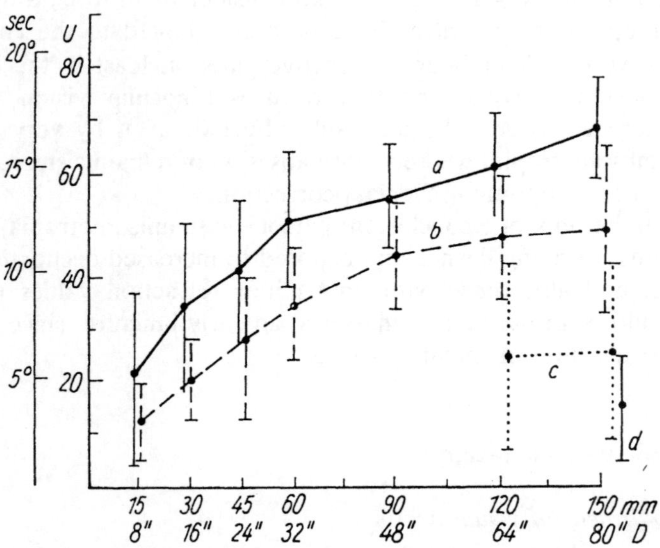

Fig. 21. Dynamic stereoacuity with standard deviation ($n = 10$) in the case of artificially induced myopic anisometropia (left eye remaining emmetropic). (*a*) Without anisometropia; (*b*) With +1.0 dpt; (*c*) +2.0 dpt; (*d*) +3.0 dpt. Abscissa: Depth distance of bars (mm), and as angle of lateral disparity (*D*). Ordinate: Revolutions per minute (right) and path in degrees per second.

affected by medium and even slight experimentally induced anisometropia. This may be due to problems resulting from the asymmetrical accommodation of the two eyes (Siebeck, 1955). The accommodation conditions of the two eyes are closely coupled to each other. Hence, sudden artificial anisometropia may cause such a large irritation of the accommodation behaviour that the more sensitive functions of binocular vision including stereoscopy are adversely affected. Severe asthenopic complaints, including cases with very low refractive differences, may result, even under natural conditions, from uncorrected anisometropia or from non-accustomed corection of natural anisometropia. Lasting anisometropia of longer persistence, however, will generally become completely integrated with the accommodation control circuit and will no longer cause any complaints or, if so, only under conditions of extreme exposures. In such cases, full correction of anisometropia would be perceived as a disturbance factor to which the binocular centres would respond by asthenopia. Such a sensitive structuring of the binocular centres may not only be seen from the susceptibility of stereoscopy to accommodation. Also, sudden alterations to one eye, for example, due to maculopathies hardly detectable by ophthalmoscopy, may quite often cause a hardly measurable reduction of visual acuity but severe impairment of binocularity, so that the patient may tend to close one eye.

Such conditions and implications are of considerable importance in everyday practice. Many individuals with anisometropia and normal vision of one eye would not use eyeglasses and would consider them to be a hinderance, since their optosensory centres have become adapted to the condition of asymmetric vision. A unilateral corrective glass, at least in the beginning, will be rejected as something that disturbs binocular vision. However, dynamic stereoscopy may be adversely affected, even by very minor uncorrected anisometropia, whereas normalisation of dynamic stereoacuity can be expected from optimum eyeglass correction.

There can be only one conclusion: persons with anisometropia, especially those holding a driving licence and exposed to increased occupational stress and strain, and also those with only minor refraction values (say, from ±1.0), should be prescribed eyeglasses at an early juncture, since this would facilitate localisation of moving objects.

6.2 Dynamic parallactoscopy

6.2.1 Impairment of visual acuity

A bar width of 7.2 mm, visible under an aperture angle of 5′30″ from a test distance of 4.5 m, was chosen to test dynamic parallactoscopy with a reduction of monocular visual acuity. General test conditions were equal to those chosen for testing dynamic stereoscopy (see Section 6.1.1). The statistical results are given in Table 7. Significant differences from normal stereoacuity were recorded from only case of 0.1 in vision.

With reasonable identifiability of the given test object, the obstruction of dynamic parallactoscopy would have to be expected only from extreme values, above all from velocities so high that dynamic visual acuity would no longer be sufficient for the clear detection of the visual object. Hence, a reduction in velocity would not have a direct effect in the form of enhanced dynamic parallactoscopy but would indirectly act via improved detection of the test object. Dynamic parallactoscopy was improved from 188″ to 112″ through a reduction of velocity from 0.5 to 0.12 m/s (see Table 7).

However, reduction of vision to $V = 0.1$ does not entail a deterioration of dynamic parallactoscopy to one-tenth of the initial value, which is likely to show the visual capability of dynamic parallactoscopy to be a sensory function of relatively high autonomy which can be reduced in performance only by factors of massive interference. The majority of people have two good or at least useful eyes. Dynamic parallactoscopy is based on perception by one eye only. Consequently, it is not at all or just negligibly affected by a reduction of visual acuity in one of these two eyes. Conditions here were found to differ substantially from those of dynamic stereoacuity which might be severely impaired by obstruction of one eye (see Section 6.1.2), since it is based on full functionality of the central systems of association which depend on impulses from both eyes. Anyhow, individuals with a merely monocular reduction of visual acuity and a properly seeing second eye would be capable, by virtue of parallactoscopy, of relatively reliable judgement of road traffic movements and would keep their three-dimensional bearings, even in difficult situations.

6.2.2 *Conditions of scotopic vision*

The luminance levels of a test surface were reduced in a stepwise manner to

Table 7. Mean values and standard deviation of three-dimensional depth at the limit of detectability from a test distance of 4.5 m, resulting from dynamic parallactoscopy (in mm and angular seconds), in cases of experimentally reduced visual acuity ($n = 10$) and at 0.5 m/s in velocity.

Visual acuity	Monocular stereoacuity	
	(mm)	(angular seconds)
1.0	15 ± 6	62 ± 24
0.6	18 ± 7	72 ± 29
0.25	18 ± 7	72 ± 29
0.1	47 ± 17	188 ± 68
0.1 and velocity of test reduced to 0.12 m/s	28 ± 10	111 ± 40

Table 8. Results recorded from investigations, using a parallactoscopometer at reduced luminance levels ($n = 10$) and at 0.5 m/s in velocity.

Luminance (cd/m^2)	Detectable average depth difference	Corresponding stereoacuity
318.9	1.5 ± 0.6	61″ ± 24″
31.9	1.4 ± 0.4	57″ ± 16″
3.2	1.6 ± 0.6	65″ ± 24″
0.3	2.7 ± 1.8	110″ ± 73″
0.06	4.6 ± 3.3	188″ ± 134″
0.03	11.6 ± 9.9	481″ ± 409″

318.9, 31.9, 3.2, 0.3, 0.06, and 0.03 cd/m^2, using a transformer connected to the lamps. The remaining test conditions were identical to those used in testing stereoacuity under conditions of scotopic vision (see Section 6.1.3).

The results obtained from those highly time-consuming investigations are summarised in Table 8. The results recorded from each of the tests involved are depicted in Fig. 22. Dynamic parallactoscopy was found to decline with surprising delay in response to a reduction of luminance, that decline not being clearly visible until a luminance level of 0.3 cd/m^2 was reached. Although Schober (1970) suggested that optimum monocular vision could no longer be attained at 31.9 cd/m^2, dynamic parallactoscopy was not reduced in performance when the luminance level of the test surface had

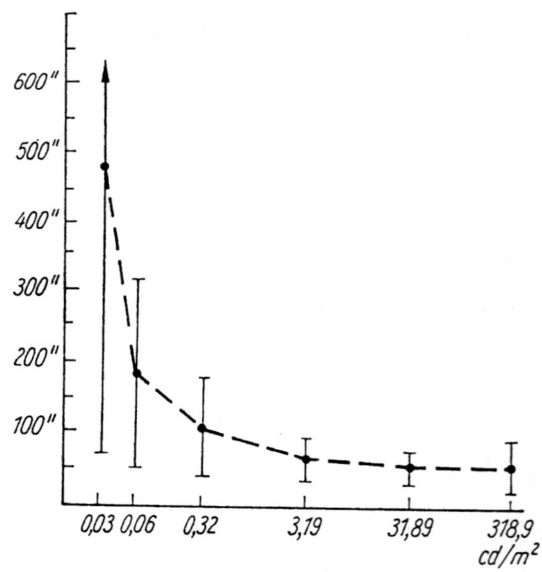

Fig. 22. Mean values and standard deviation of dynamic parallactic stereoacuity in response to reduced luminance levels ($n = 10$). Abscissa: Luminance (cd/m^2). Ordinate: Stereoacuity in angular seconds (″).

been reduced from 620 cd/m^2 at the beginning to 31.9 cd/m^2. Evaluable three-dimensional information was obtainable from movement parallax, even at a luminance level of 0.03 cd/m^2, a value at which stereoscopic perception should only be possible in very rare cases (see Section 6.1.1). A remarkable amount of dynamic parallactoscopy, which might be considerably helpful in three-dimensional orientation in every-day life, continued to exist under conditions of scotopic vision down to 0.06 cd/m^2 in luminance. Dynamic parallactoscopy was quite obviously less strongly impaired by unsafe fixation and inhibited oculomotoricity, due to scotopia which has a detrimental impact upon stereoscopy, and it appeared to be just as negligibly affected by dark mydriasis and nocturnal myopia. After all, binocular fusion, taking a much longer time with reduced luminance than with light adaptation (Piper, 1951), would not be necessary for monocular movement parallax.

Identical or similar findings may be assumed for the majority of the other empirical factors of three-dimensional perception, primarily for the appraisal of size ratios, linear perspective, and an overlapping of contours.

7. Effect of psychosensorial factors

Sophisticated sensomotor performance, including dynamic stereoscopy, has been proved, by experience, to depend to a considerable extent on the psychic condition of a human being. For a long time, this has been taken into due consideration in sports, occupational activities, and other spheres of life. A decline in static stereoacuity, similar to that caused by physical stress or sleep deficit, was observed by Heinsius (1944) in situations of high psychical stress.

Stereoscopic vision was found to depend on numerous intricate associations in the central nervous system together with psychological dependencies. In the twenties, there were good reasons for psychologists to pay great attention to problems relating to stereoscopic vision and for making substantial contributions to them. However, the position of the mind had continuously been the subject of controversial views and discussions, quite different from the physiological foundations of stereoscopic vision, above all stereoscopy in the form of lateral disparity (Krudewig, 1953; Mayer, 1977). Physiologists used to take remarkably reserved attitudes to the teachings and reasoning of psychology. A full account of psychological aspects relating to all levels of stereoscopy was given by Linschoten (1956) in a comprehensive monograph.

Some importance should be attributed, in this context, to the findings recorded from psychiatric patients who had been examined for binocular vision. Stereoscopic findings recorded by Krause and Hempel (1982) from cases of paranoic schizophrenia, catatonic schizophrenia, hebephrenic schizophrenia, and schizoaffective syndrome (cycloidism), as well as from cases of depressive and maniacal syndromes or of cerebro-organic lesions, and even from cases of minor psychic disorders, were less significant than the values obtained from normal persons, with illusionary perceptions having been ruled out beforehand. Peculiarities of creative expression of psychiatric patients with regard to three-dimensionality were analysed in great detail by Rennert (1977). He established organically and functionally caused alterations to three-dimensional patterns as well as to three-dimensionality of perception and reproduction, with deficits in perception being measurable by means of sensorial physiology and ophthalmology. Similar results were reported by Kienle (1968), E. and G. Schulz (1974), and Wäldrich (1978). Their findings produced evidence to the effect that, in cases of impaired sensomotor coordination, loss of attentiveness, and inadequacy of transformation, CNS-dependent processing of two- or three-dimensional impressions was possible only in an atypical or psychopathological manner or was not possible at all, with particular attention being paid to effects of neuroleptic and antidepressive agents upon binocular sensomotoricity (Toppel, 1976).

Dynamic stereoscopy implies a combination of stereoscopy with oculomotoricity, the latter being highly irritated by psychic aspects. It, therefore, seems to be quite opportune to try to analyse at least some of those psychic factors that are accessible for experimental studies.

7.1 Fatigue

Fatigue is associated to a great deal with psychic phenomena, which plays a substantial role in all tests relating to sophisticated movements or measurements of sensory performance. This fully applies to the determination of dynamic stereoacuity. It is almost impossible for a test person to optimally concentrate on any given process without interruption for an extended period of time and to give such high-continuity attention to a complete test programme. Fatigue tends to manifest itself in two ways, as a psychosomatic phenomenon or in the form of what is called psychic saturation.

Early onset of fatigue is a widespread disorder which may quite correctly be defined as a disease. Cerebral activity is modified under conditions of fatigue. Stronger stimulae and even high-intensity impulses for attentiveness may quite often be processed in the normal way. Fatigue may have psychogenic but also organic, constitutional, functional, and exogenic causes. Severe fatigue due to mental or physical overtaxing may entail impairment of retinal blood circulation. According to Schober (1972), this might result in the perception of whitish spots in the visual field or minor scotomas, with those visual field defects not even deliberately perceived. Pupils are somewhat dilated under conditions of fatigue. This may slighly reduce visual acuity and was found to be conducive to asthenopia, epiphora, and vulnerability to glare in over 25 percent of all probands examined for such phenomena (Kiriyakoff, Vassileva and Raicheva, 1964). Dubois-Poulsen (1968), on the other hand, observed, within the context of fatigue, that it was merely a disorder of oculomotoricity rather than an impairment of sensoricity.

The term 'psychic saturation' (Jaensch, 1939) was closely associated with fatigue. According to his findings, this kind of reduction in performance originated from the long-time stereotypic action of one and the same stimulus on the sense of a test person. Such adverse effects might be supported by indifference or uncritical attitude towards one's own capabilities. In long-distance car driving, this might lead to an underestimation of distance and speed or delayed reaction to difficult traffic situations. That is why a three-dimensional impression tends to be gradually flattened when a depth distance is watched for an extended length of time.

A number of observations have already become known regarding the impact of fatigue on stereoscopic vision. Heinsius (1947) examined naval range-finders after a nightwatch, strenuous sea voyage, and psychic stress, and found their stereopsis substantively reduced, especially at night. Leopoldsberger (1942) observed substantial impairment of fusion in soldiers after three hours of drill which was further aggravated after the intake of alcohol. Similar findings were reported by Giardini (1949). R. Sachsenweger (1955) found fatigue to affect stereopsis, primarily after the repeated momentary presentation of a test object and in mesopic vision, yet with wide-ranging variations. The time needed to generate a three-dimensional impression was found to increase along with fatigue.

The degree of fatigue, unfortunately, cannot be reliably determined by means of physiological or psychotechnical tests. This, on the other hand, is not absolutely essential for the verification of dynamic vision, since fatigue is generally expressed in many and variable ways by almost all persons tested, beyond any normal measure of inter-individual scatter. This is characterised, for example, by growing error rates or subjective perception of indifference.

The factor of fatigue was considered to be important enough, under ergophthalmological aspects, to analyse its relevance to dynamic stereoacuity. For that reason, three probands were subjected to dynamic stereoacuity testing for 90 min without interruption and close to threshold levels. Fairly considerable demands were made in those test programmes on both stereoscopic optosensoricity and oculomotoricity. They were approximately equivalent to 60 km of downtown driving or 150 km of highway driving at high speeds. All test persons were chosen to be above 55 years of age, since it was well known that individuals of advanced ages were likely to be struck by fatigue sooner and more severely than younger persons. After 90 min, or even earlier, all test persons more or less exhibited massive symptoms of fatigue along with an unambiguous drop in performance, although they had been warned in advance and briefed on the project and the intention to test for fatigue and concentration after lasting stress on dynamic stereopsis. It could not be ruled out that the peculiarity of the test situation had, at least to some extent, stimulated their concentration. Dynamic stereoacuity dropped by about 30 percent in a woman aged 55 years and by 25 percent in another woman of 63 and even by half the original vision in a male proband of 67. Original levels were restored after a break of 5 min.

Fatigue is highly variable in the context of dynamic stereopsis. Genuine failures have usually occurred in response to massive overtaxing, as has been also reported for static stereoacuity or binocular fusion by Dubois-Poulsen (1969) and Leopoldsberger (1942).

The task of making a specific performance through cooperation between the two eyes, which would not be feasible by means of monocular vision, must necessarily lead to overtaxing and, thus, premature fatigue. This is of relevance to occupational medicine, in that it offers an explanation for frequent visual problems in the context of those activities which call for permanent or predominant three-dimensional observation and appraisal. It might also explain the phenomenon of wishing to close one eye in an attempt to cope with fatigue resulting from permanent binocular strain. The visual process may thus be changed to monocular vision, which is possible with much lower associative effort, though stereoscopy would be renounced altogether.

Impairment of dynamic stereoacuity may, possibly, provoke fatigue in its own right, since with reduced dynamic stereoscopy, any kind of visual perception would make higher demands on individual performance potential and would, thus, lead to premature fatigue.

Fatigue, in connection with dynamic parallactoscopy, was found to be much lower than that associated with dynamic stereoscopy. It was also found to be reduced to individually variable subjective perception of overtaxing or lack of interest, without resulting in unambiguous signs of lowered performance. Prolongation of exercise periods had to be abandoned for external reasons. The less demanding but more reflectory setup of dynamic parallactoscopy and its much less complicated nature, were underlined by the fact that kinetoparallactic vision was accompanied by a much lower predisposition to fatigue. The threshold of fatigue was obviously equal to that of elementary vision. Secondary factors, such as physical constitution prior to exposure to stress and psychic condition, were presumably just as important to test results as the repetition of end-of-test demands.

7.2 Effect of psychosedatives

There is a sizeable number of people taking psychopharmaceuticals in the form of psychosedatives and still actively participating in road traffic. Many of them are additionally exposed to the risk of industrial accident at their places of work or as pedestrians in high-density urban traffic. Psychosedatives (minor tranquillisers, ataractics) which were introduced into the therapy for non-specific attenuation of anxiety in 1952, are really capable of manipulating psychic processes but, at the same time, tend to cause a strongly pronounced decrease of reactivity. Similar considerations would apply to the majority of neuroleptics (major tranquillisers, antipsychotics). There are only a few psychopharmaceuticals which have a direct action on the eyes or ocular muscles, e.g. on accommodation, sensitivity to dazzling or visual acuity, perhaps as a result of chorioretinopathy, pupillomotoricity, field of vision, dark adaptation, colour perception, and time of retinal conduction (Lieschke, 1982).

While psychopharmaceuticals will rarely cause direct impairment of the visual capacity, they are likely to affect the personality as a whole, together with psychomotoricity, and may, consequently, lead to poor road conduct (Gramberg-Danielsen, 1976). Psychopharmaceuticals are likely to affect, with high probability, associative processes in the central nervous system and, consequently, the very bases of dynamic stereoacuity. They are thus capable of stimulating in a decisive way all performances of the central nervous system (Schmidt, 1983).

Faustan® (5 mg of diazepam in one tablet) is a very common psycho-sedative and, therefore, was chosen from among the psychopharmaceuticals to test its effects upon dynamic stereoacuity and dynamic parallactoscopy. Dynamic stereoacuity was determined prior to administration of two tablets of Faustan® and one hour after intake.

Remarkable individual differences were recorded regarding the intensity of the Faustan® action. It had almost soporific effects on some persons and almost no palpable effects on others, so that all stages between maximum and minimum tranquillisation were noticed. Inter-individual blood-level scatter was between 1:10 and 1:30, despite body-weight related dosage (Walter, Uchtländer and Meyer, 1983).

None of the six probands exhibited any effect, a result so unambiguous that the experiment was discontinued after the sixth person had been tested.

Such a result, however, could not entirely rule out a possible impact of the pharmaceutical on dynamic stereoacuity in certain extraordinary cases, for example, in conjunction with the intake of low quantities of alcohol generating very low blood-alcohol levels or after psychic overtaxing and the lack of sleep, etc. Nevertheless, these proved to be factors which were hardly accessible to experimental analysis. By no means should the conclusion be drawn from the above negative findings that warning patients against medication and driving was overcautious and, consequently, unnecessary. Also, when either type of dynamic stereoacuity was tested, high attentiveness and concentration were required for only a few seconds. There was no surprise element in the test room and no source of exhaustion, with optosensoricity being confronted with optimum conditions of vision.

A totally different situation will face an individual while driving a car. Visibility will quite often be close to the threshold of control. Attentiveness will be required in all parts of the visual field and not only for the gaze ahead. There will be a permanent compulsion towards ocular movements. With almost no pause for reflection, there will be ever new demands on vision, resulting from changing road traffic situations. A driver's attention might also be diverted by passengers or radio programmes or the tiring monotony of the road. In a real situation, all these factors might considerably suppress dynamic stereoacuity of a person on psychosedatives, so that failure could not be ruled out. According to Schott and Seidel (1982), misgivings regarding driving fitness might be unjustified in cases of long-time low-dosage psychopharmaceutical therapy, if no side effects with relevance to road safety medicine were detectable. This might be helpful to medical examiners in taking the appropriate driving fitness decisions on probands under such therapeutic regimes, depending on individual clinical pictures.

There can be no doubt about the severe depression of dynamic vision by psychotropic drugs (Gramberg-Danielsen, 1976). Hashish, for example, has no effect on visual acuity nor on colour vision, but has clearly pronounced consequences for all forms of stereoscopic vision (Helmer, 1972).

Opposite effects were found to result from analeptics, above all, when these were taken under the conditions of fatigue and exhaustion. Many studies had been conducted particulary into caffeine and its effects on visual functions, though with contradictory results. For example, cases were reported of improvement in contrast perception, lower sensitivity to dazzling, enhancement of scotopic vision, reduced time of re-adaptation, and ERG changes (Gramberg-Danielsen, 1976). Coffee was found to have stimulating effects on the majority of people for only about 30 min, followed by a deceleration of reactivity, with a few exceptions, which had calming effects. Tea, on the other hand, proved to be less vehement in action, but the stimulating effects were thought to last for two to three hours.

7.3 Effect of hypnotics

Great importance, in terms of occupational and transport medicine, should also be attributed to the variability of visual capacity in response to the intake of hypnotics. A generally increasing consumption of soporifics has been accompanied by the growing number of people in whom medicinal effects had not worn off the next morning on their way to work. Hypnotics were found to act primarily on three components of eye functionality, external oculomotoricity, binocular functions, and pupillomotoricity (Gramberg-Danielsen, 1976).

Barbiturates appeared to be less suitable for the following series of experiments, since they primarily stimulated vegetative centres along the limiting line between mesencephalon and diencephalon and, consequently, had only secondary effects upon cerebral centres and pathways, consciousness, reactivity, impulse receptivity, and evaluation of stimuli.

Fatigue was induced by the simultaneous intake of two tablets of Dormutil® (200 mg of methaqualone per tablet). Yet, the examiners very soon found that the resulting fatigue could be offset at any time for the duration of the testing through particular attentiveness efforts. In the tests, the above-mentioned six persons did not exhibit any significant difference between dynamic stereoacuity and dynamic parallactoscopy prior to and one hour after administration of the soporific. A substantial role had been played, no doubt, by dosage. A performance-depressive effect would eventually occur in response to overdosage.

Hence, when it comes to endurance activities, such as driving, etc., impairment of dynamic stereoacuity in response to soporifics should be expected, notwithstanding the above negative results. It cannot be ruled out, on the other hand, that even after pharmaceutically induced fatigue, failure will not occur, since no difficult situation was encountered during the day.

A study into the effect of alcohol on dynamic stereoacuity could be unnecessary, since other authors have safely established in the past that blood alcohol levels as low as 0.3 percent (equivalent to 0.3 g of alcohol to 1 kg of body weight) would have an adverse impact upon monocular dynamic visual acuity (Honegger, Kampfschulte and Klein, 1972; Kühner, 1958). Those effects were found to be primarily generated by impairment of oculomotoricity rather than by direct action on the sensorial system, particularly as ethyl alcohol proved to weaken attentiveness, reactivity, concentration, and gaze control (Gramberg-Danielsen, 1976), but was of relatively minor relevance to visual acuity, stereoacuity, width of fusion (Manz, 1939), and colour vision. Alcohol-related alterations to sensorial performance were primarily noticed under unfavourable lighting conditions (Gramberg-Danielsen, 1976). The reaction to alcohol of dynamic stereoacuity and dynamic parallactoscopy may be expected to be identical to the reaction of monocular dynamic visual acuity.

7.4 Short-time and long-time exercises

Practice is a relevant factor in vision at all levels. It has proved to be of particular importance in children and adolescents and in persons with visual defects. It was found to be less feasible for visual performance by individuals of advanced age (van Beuningen, 1949). Consideration of the effects of exercise is absolutely essential in repetitive ophthalmological examinations lest the examiner should be trapped by illusionary improvement.

Due consideration should also be given to the effects of exercise and practice in ophthalmological research, if false conclusions are to be avoided. Therefore, it would be advisable to have the actual recording and documentation of findings preceded by a phase of exercises. Five to 10 settings should be sufficient to cover 90 percent of the exercise effect in the context of dynamic monocular visual acuity (Honegger, Kampfschulte and Klein, 1970; Honegger, Schaefer and Jaeger, 1969; Ludvigh and Miller, 1958).

There is, no doubt, a long-time exercise effect, as well. Static stereoacuity continued to improve up to the 13th day of the exercise, according to Haberkorn (1965). However, inter-individual variations could not be offset by exercise (Rüssel, 1939). Van Beuningen (1949) observed long-time effects in the second and third weeks, after daily measurements, depending, however, on the types of testing instruments used. Enormous inter-individual scatter, depending on intelligence, education, concentration, constitution, age, and other factors, had to be reckoned with in the context of both short- and long-time exercise effects.

A binocular rotational prismometer was used on three persons being tested to measure dynamic stereoacuity on some 20 consecutive days, followed by longer intervals (over six weeks altogether). The probands were of similar age and included two females aged 54 and 62 years and one male aged 67, so that a substantive age-related effect could be widely ruled out. Several days of testing showed that a major increase in results could not be expected, implying that the testing method chosen had no or only very minor long-time exercise effects. A short-time exercise effect, however, was clearly detectable. Results recorded from 10 persons at the beginning (after briefing and after 10 tentative settings) were compared to those recorded after some 80 additional settings. The average exercise effect on the 10 persons is given in Fig. 23. Significance calculation revealed a difference between the two curves with an error probability of 0.1 percent.

Several practicable factors are likely to have a coordinated effect when it comes to dynamic stereoacuity: static visual acuity, static stereoacuity,

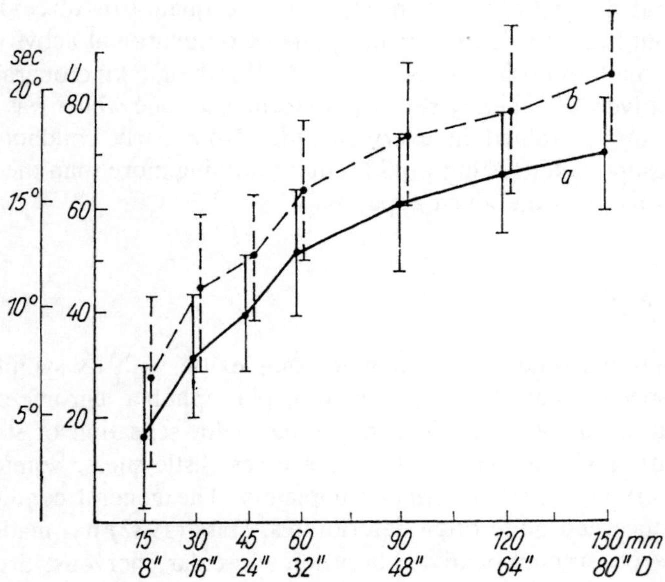

Fig. 23. Mean values and standard deviation of dynamic stereoacuity ($n = 10$) at start of testing (*a*) and after another 80 settings (*b*) to determine short-time exercise effect. Abscissa: Depth distance of bars (mm), and as angle of lateral disparity (*D*). Ordinate: Revolutions per minute (right) and path in degrees per second.

dynamic visual acuity, and oculomotoricity with its capability of fixation and pursuit movements. Static visual acuity was found to be the only one of these factors with a relatively narrow range of scatter of the exercise effect. The multiplicity of practicable factors, as a whole, has proved to yield a wide-ranging variety of exercise results.

Using a triple-bar apparatus, van Beuningen (1949) recorded from the following different modes of reaction of static stereoacuity to repetitive exercises: (1) test persons with good and constant stereoscopic performance, (2) test persons with moderate performance and good exercise results, (3) test persons with initially poor performance which was elevated by exercises to moderate levels, (4) test persons with poor performance and large scatter of exercise results, and (5) test persons with inadequate stereoscopic performance which could hardly be enhanced by exercise.

A good routine method for ophthalmological practice should ensure that an initial exercise effect did not exceed 25 percent of the initial value and that the results should become relatively constant after four to five days. This demand is met by both the rotational prismometer and parallactoscopometer.

An exercise effect was no longer recordable by the parallactoscopometer after the tenth setting, and, in most cases, even before the tenth setting. The short-time exercise effect was negligible in all probands, and a long-time exercise effect was not recordable at all. This is in agreement with the insight that a significant enhancement in the quality of three-dimensional vision would not result from many years of occupational activity with high demands on stereopsis (see Section 4.3.2) and that kinetoparallactoscopy was a relatively elementary sensory performance, one which was intensively but unwittingly trained in every-day life, from early childhood, so that parallactosopometer testing would require nothing more than the adaptation of the proband to the given apparatus.

7.5 Asthenopia

The asthenopia syndrome is of high complexity, with its symptoms being quite unspecific, but including epiphora, photophobia, chronic conjunctivitis, sensation of light flashes in the visual field, sensation of stress on the eyes, blurred vision, nausea in severe cases, listlessness, vomiturition, as well as nervous gastro-intestinal complaints. The general condition of the person concerned quite often deteriorates. Hass (1982) has made a distinction between accommodative (dioptric), muscular, nervous, artificial, and environment-related forms of asthenopia. The causative abnormality may quite often be of no substantial magnitude and, therefore, may be unnoticed in routine diagnosis. Vision is particularly impaired by asymmetries between the two eyes (see Section 6.1.2). Asthenopic complaints may also occur in concomitance with liability of binocular vision (de Decker and Haase, 1976; Otto and Höllmüller, 1969).

Visuosensorial or oculomotoric stresses of a specific nature are usually involved in the development and manifestation of asthenopia. Almost every case of asthenopia reflects a discrepancy between visual capability and demand on vision. Consequently, asthenopia is of a situation-specific nature and usually manifests itself only under certain circumstances. Impaired resistance may be a consequence of systemic neurodystonia. The incidence of asthenopia was found to be highly variable in different populations (Schober, 1954), depending on occupational activities, general stresses and strains, and ways of life.

It cannot be ruled out that asthenopia can be provoked by reduced dynamic stereoacuity, especially as the incidence of asthenopia was found to be higher in quite a number of occupational activities for which dynamic stereoacuity was more often demanded than elsewhere. Therefore, 10 persons with a reported history of asthenopic complaints were examined for dynamic stereoscopy, and eight comparable probands were checked for dynamic parallactoscopy. All probands were without contributory ophthalmological findings. None of them was suffering asthenopic complaints at the time of testing. No statistically significant difference was found to exist for both modes of stereopsis between these probands, on the one hand, and probands involved in a mass screening programme, on the other. Four persons reported that their asthenopic complaints usually arose during long periods of motorcar driving, an activity which is dominated by movement vision and exposed to increased demands on dynamic stereoacuity. Dynamic stereoacuity in these four persons was normal and, consequently, had to be ruled out as a cause of asthenopia.

8. Comparison between dynamic and kinetoparallactic stereoacuities

The following may be clearly seen from plotting threshold values of dynamic stereoscopy together with those of dynamic parallactoscopy on the same diagram: While dynamic stereoscopy provides highly precise and detailed three-dimensional orientation, it tends to fail in response to even moderate velocities. The visual result of dynamic parallactoscopy would be less precise and detailed, but would be relatively independent of velocity and would thus ensure much better three-dimensional orientation, even in response to high velocities. Dynamic stereoscopy was found to be about three times more efficient than dynamic parallactoscopy in the context of low velocities. Both were identical to one another, say, for slow pedestrian speeds. The effectiveness of either stereoscopic function was clearly narrowed in response to an artificial reduction of visual acuity, although such a narrowing was less than expected in response to a more drastic reduction of visual acuity and was by no means parallel to the latter. Dynamic parallactoscopy, quite different from dynamic stereoscopy, remained intact for relatively extended periods of time, after a drastic reduction of luminance levels.

The interaction of stereoscopy with movement parallactoscopy and the inter-relationship between these two, are of great importance for all practical purposes. A comparison can be helpful in determining the point at which dynamic stereoscopy, together with dynamic stereoacuity, constitutes the decisive upper limit of performance or the point at which that upper limit is determined by dynamic parallactoscopy together with kinetoparallactic stereoacuity, or at what levels a visual performance would be insufficient or would be complementary to another. This is of particular importance in situations in which either mode of visual performance may be impaired by inhibitory factors, such as reduced visual acuity or twilight.

An analysis will now be made of visual performance resulting from dynamic stereoacuity on the basis of positional parallax of both eyes as a function of stereoscopy, on the one hand, and of stereoacuity on the basis of the additionally possible monocular movement parallax as a function of kinetoparallactic stereopsis, on the other. Other forms of stereopsis were found to be important only in certain defined cases but, such cases are decisive in accuracy in comparison to both dynamic stereoscopy as well as dynamic parallactoscopy.

However, comparison between dynamic stereoacuity and kinetoparallactic stereoacuity would not be easily possible under sensorial aspects, since the thresholds of these two forms of perception would be determined by totally different sensory qualities. Nevertheless, a comparison of that kind would be in compliance with numerous everyday requirements, above all in the context of occupational fitness, criteria for expert opinions, elucidation of causes of accidents, etc.

Compensation for highly variable test conditions is likely to be the most difficult task in such a comparison. Dynamic stereoacuity, for example, has to be determined in circular movement, whereas dynamic parallactic stereoacuity must be measured in linear movement. Results recorded by Honegger, Schaefer and Jaeger (1969) for dynamic visual acuity from a linear presentation of optotypes were four times better than those obtained from optotypes in circular movement. That relationship was only approximate and was determined only for dynamic visual acuity, but it probably seems to be applicable to all forms of movement vision. The thresholds of dynamic stereoacuity were, therefore, corrected by a factor of four.

The two functions of stereopsis are figuratively compared to each other in the semi-diagrammatic Figs. 24 to 27, with some important differences being revealed between them. The area which can be three-dimensionally assessed

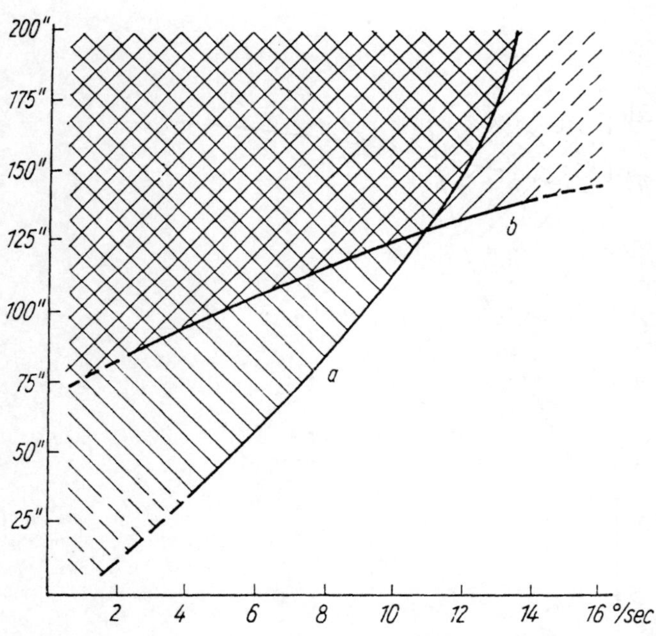

Fig. 24. Semi-diagram of levels of dynamic stereoscopy (mean value curve *a*) and dynamic parallactoscopy (mean value curve *b*) under optimum visual conditions. Cross-hatched perceivable by either type of stereopsis; non-hatched area not perceivable by either type. Abscissa: Path in degrees per second (see Table 5). Ordinate: Stereoacuity in angular (″).

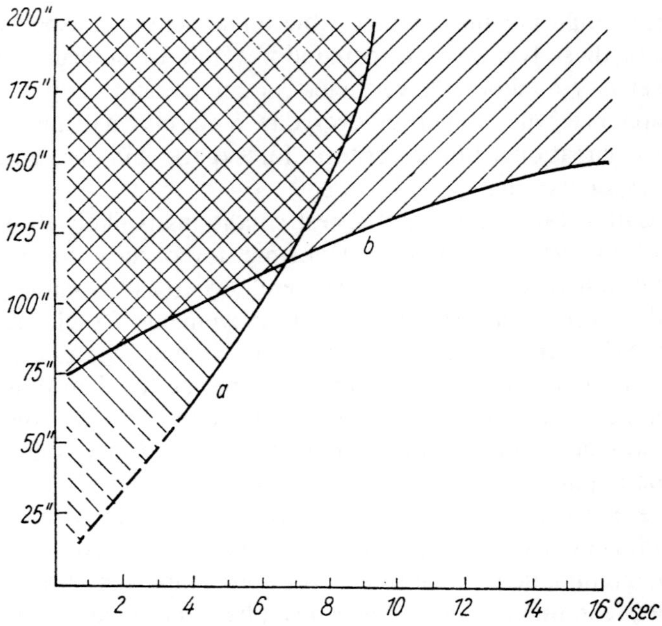

Fig. 25. Same as Fig. 24, but with visual acuity reduced to $V = 0.25$.

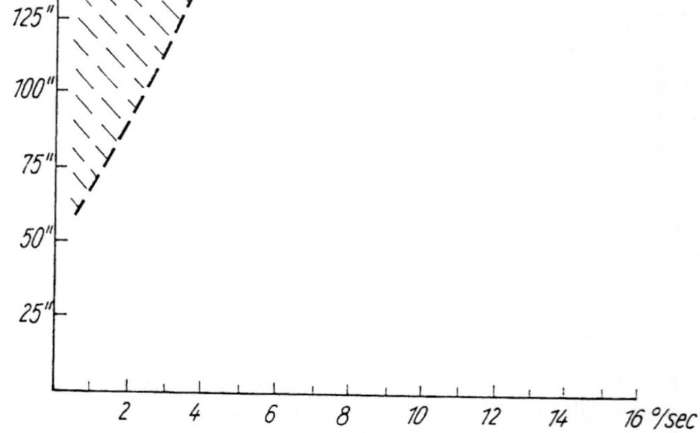

Fig. 26. Same as Fig. 24, but with visual acuity experimentally reduced to $V = 0.1$.

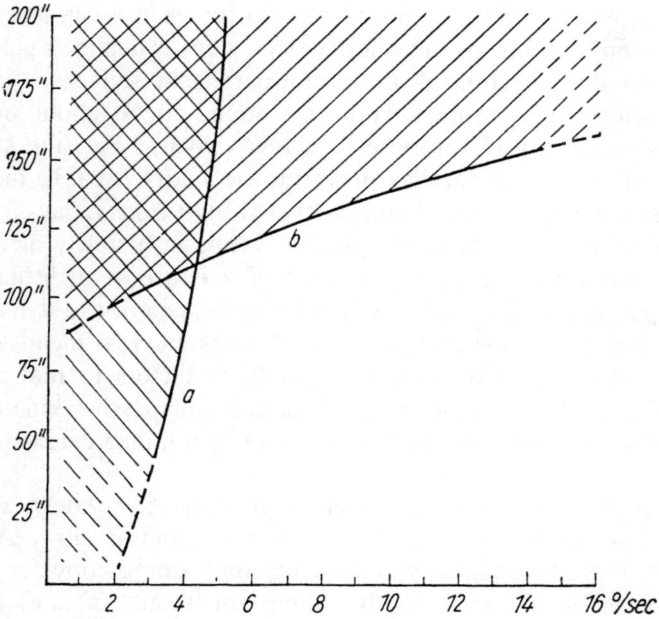

Fig. 27. Same as Fig. 24, but with luminance reduced to 0.3 cd/m².

by both functions (two different forms of dynamic visual perception), has been line-hatched. The stereoscopically perceivable area (above and left from curve *a*) provides for a considerably accurate stereopsis of between 10″ and 75″ (i.e. a depth distance of something between 20 and 130 mm, from a test distance of 5 m), but only for relatively slow-moving visual objects (Fig. 24). With larger three-dimensional distances, the area of dynamic parallactic vision is superimposed on the stereoscopically perceivable area, but reveals a much wider and more comprehensive effectiveness in performance with velocities of some 14 °/sec (about 1.25 m/s or 4.5 km/h, from a test distance of 5 m).

An area which continuously increases in size in response to an increase in velocity is situated left below and right from the two curves. Here, three-dimensional localisation is not possible, neither on the basis of dynamic stereoscopy nor on the basis of subjective movement parallactoscopy, since vision is two-dimensional unless three-dimensional perception becomes possible due to the involvement of other factors, e.g., those related to experience. The area in which either form of perception is possible (cross-hatched) may be seen to grow in size along with growing differences in distances among targets and in spite of higher velocities.

Dynamic stereoacuity has been shown to depend strongly on velocity, a fact that cannot be simply explained by the decline in visual acuity in response to moving objects (see Section 2.1). An indecisive role, on the other hand, was found to be played by velocity when it came to movement parallactoscopy, as long as the velocity-dependent dynamic visual acuity was sufficient for the detection of object and parallactic shift.

The efficiency of parallactoscopy was found to be about one-third of dynamic stereoacuity in response to a low velocity. Yet, the stereoscopic threshold of movement parallax proved to be nearly equal to the threshold of stereoscopic depth acuity, along with a rising velocity, say, from 10 °/sec (comparable to slow pedestrian speeds). Sitting in a slowly driven car and watching, while moving past, the front of a house at a distance of 5 m, dynamic parallactoscopy will clearly begin to be superior to dynamic stereoscopy. When the car speeds up, the depth assessment by means of parallactoscopy, will be superior by a multiplicity of factors to that assessed by means of dynamic stereoscopy, with active and passive kinetoparallactic stereoacuity differing from each other only to a minor extent (see Section 4.2.1).

Detailed three-dimensional orientation may be widely ensured by dynamic stereoscopy, as long as target movement is slow. Accuracy of stereopsis is predominantly based on dynamic stereoscopy for lateral disparities of up to 75″ (i.e. depth distance of about 130 mm, from a test distance of 5 m). Kinetoparallactic stereoacuity was proved to be more effective than dynamic stereoscopy at 125″ (i.e. depth distance of about 35 mm, from a test distance of 5 m and a 40 cm observation pathway), as long as properly visible test objects are used. Yet, dynamic stereoacuity under every-day conditions of visual requirements is probably better than in a bar test, as may be seen from tests where two depth-distant surfaces had been used (see Section 5.1.6).

Substantial displacement of magnitudes has been observed under conditions of reduced visual acuity and reduced luminance levels. Increasingly growing areas were recordable with three-dimensional perception no longer being possible, with stereoscopy being more severely impaired than dynamic parallactoscopy.

Kinetoparallactic stereopsis was found to remain approximately constant in comparison to unaffected visual acuity, when the latter was $V = 0.25$ (Fig. 25). Dynamic stereoacuity, however, was already clearly reduced at that point. Kinetoparallactic stereopsis was found to be strongly narrowed when visual acuity had come down to $V = 0.1$ (Fig. 26), without dynamic stereoacuity being substantially worsened. In every-day visual activity, with decreasing visual acuity and clear visibility of targets and slow velocity, the predominance of dynamic stereoscopy in the perception of low-depth distances was found to be remarkably persistent.

The range within which stereoscopic vision is possible tends to shrink considerably in response to the reduction of luminance to 0.3 cd/m^2, i.e. just before scotopia, whereas hardly any limitations in performance are exhibited by dynamic parallactoscopy (Fig. 27).

9. Conclusions

Relatively little parallelism was found to exist between still and moving objects with regard to three-dimensional vision. Hence, additional dynamic vision testing may be necessary. This is true for both dynamic stereoscopy and dynamic parallactoscopy. The binocular rotational prismometer or parallactoscopometer proved to be highly suitable for testing within that context. There are specific situations in transport, occupational, and sports medicines in which stereoacuity should be tested in conjunction with oculomotoricity, taking into due consideration the inseparable physiological links between the two.

There are plenty of three-dimensional movements in the human environment and particularly on road traffic, and proper visual perception of movement can be of crucial importance to job performance and to the rate of traffic accidents although systematic studies have not so far been conducted into the stereoscopic pursuit of moving objects. Vision and movement are closely associated with each other. Yet, the movement factor has so far been blotted out, on grounds of practicability, from all investigations on visual power. Still objects were used as optotypes in vision tests, which meant the rejection of job-related and traffic-related analysis.

There is no parallelism at all between the vision of still and moving objects. Evidence to that effect has been produced by early studies into monocular dynamic visual acuity (Ludvigh and Miller, 1958; Jaeger and Honegger, 1964). Individuals with good static visual acuity do not necessarily possess good dynamic visual capacity. This is a decisive aspect, no doubt, when it comes to the appraisal of fitness for certain occupational activities. The same applies to dynamic stereoacuity.

Dynamic three-dimensional vision is based on two optosensorial capabilities, binocular stereoscopy and movement parallactoscopy or kinetoparallactoscopy, the latter also being possible in a monocular manner. Dynamic stereopsis can be properly measured by means of the recently developed binocular rotational prismometer (see Section 3.1). Its enormous precision has the greatest effect at short distances (not more than 10 m). When it comes to longer distances, vision was found to be more strongly determined by empirical factors of three-dimensional perception and was found to be decisively determined by dynamic parallactoscopy (seeing moving objects on the basis of movement parallax). The latter can be effectively measured by means of a recently devised parallactoscopometer (see Section 3.2).

Dynamic stereoacuity is a highly subtle and remarkably sophisticated sensorial achievement of sensitive reactivity. It is based on stereoscopy, binocular fixation, motor and sensory fusion, and the capability of ocular pursuit movement. These basic factors are highly variable, even in normally sighted individuals. Dynamic stereoacuity is characterised by wide variability. However, stereoscopy has its limits, some of them depending on the associative performance of the central nervous system through which two-dimensional images of lateral disparity are transformed to a three-dimensional perception on the retinae of the two eyes.

On the basis of movement parallax, i.e. dynamic parallactoscopy, stereopsis has been the phylogenetically earlier and, consequently, more stable visual capacity by which to perceive a three-dimensional situation. Its sensorial accuracy has proved to be very much below that of dynamic stereoscopy in response to slow velocities. But it has been found to assume an absolutely predominant position in response to moderate and high velocities. It is largely based on the capability of fixation in the course of ocular pursuit movement and, if one eye is visually reduced, on the monocular visual acuity or visual acuity of the better eye.

These two components of three-dimensional vision and their sensorial capabilities, are not just of interest from the ophthalmological and sensophysiological points of view. They are certainly of particular relevance to occupational and transport medicine. The visual demands made by quite a number of activities and occupations have grown considerably in relation to technological progress (Merte, 1978), and the need is growing for the formulation of specific criteria of occupational fitness, primarily regarding dynamic stereopsis. This particular need had been left unconsidered in almost all national and international programmes of occupational fitness rating, especially in terms of performance-related and methodological rules or regulations (Broschmann, 1981). Stereoacuity for the perception of moving objects should become part of eye testing for quite a number of activities.

Any reduction of dynamic stereoacuity may lead to inadequate visual information and may, thus, assume a straightforward relevance to occupational and transport medicine. Individuals who fail to achieve normal performance in three-dimensional orientation are, in a way, handicapped from the very outset, since, in certain situations, they may be unable to do their jobs according to safety regulations or machine specifications.

Motorcar driving ranks high among the practice-related aspects of dynamic stereoacuity. Stereoscopically sighted individuals who suddenly become monocular, may lose a great deal of security in road traffic, e.g., in slow convoy driving, pulling into parking gaps, reversing, assessment of short distances, driving on lanes narrowed by parked vehicles, turning into gateways, or overtaking (Aulhorn, 1976). True, there is something like age-dependent gradual adjustment to monocularity (Heydenreich and Wittwer, 1981), which, however, is no substitute for the loss of stereoscopic vision. On the other hand, persons who have turned monocular are at little or no disadvantage at all in moving traffic. Good stereoscopic vision of road traffic is essential within a range of up to 20 m (Broschmann, 1981; Hartmann and Stöcker, 1983). Piper (1969) found stereoscopy to be highly important up to 50 m, Heinsius (1964) even up to 90 m. Yet, stereoscopic impressions will become unevaluable for practical purposes, if visual targets are located at long distances from the observer.

Three-dimensional perception of moving processes in road traffic travelling at high speeds is ensured by movement parallax. It is an advantage in road traffic that the most important objects of observation, other vehicles, are also moving, which provides for the summation of several three-dimensional impressions. In road traffic, stereoscopic vision is simply a complementary, though not unimportant sensorial security (Dubois-Poulsen, 1969; Schumann, 1959; Broschmann, 1977, 1981). Finally, inadequate dynamic stereoscopy is likely to have consequences in terms of driving economy due to less calm and more nervous driving, resulting in too frequent deceleration or acceleration.

A train driver, on the other hand, would only have to concentrate on objects straight ahead, so that, to him, dynamic stereoacuity plays an absolutely subordinate role. Again, this does not apply to train drivers involved in shunting (Vesper, 1965).

Stereoscopic vision is not absolutely imperative for aircraft pilots. They have to deal exclusively with fast movement and long distances for which kinetoparallactic vision was found to be more important than stereoscopy (Epstein and Tredici, 1973). Accordingly, no insufficiencies were displayed by professional or amateur pilots who had been blindfolded on one eye. Hence, stereoscopy may be rated as some kind of 'luxurious' asset to flyers (Aichmair, 1983; Grosslight, Fletscher, Masterton and Hagen, 1978). However, Mayer and Lane (1973) found that the number of monocular pilots involved in near or actual accidents had been higher than that of pilots with intact stereoscopy. Sport and glider pilots, parachutists, and helicopter pilots, on the other hand, were found to depend strongly on the accurate assessment of moving objects and, thus, on dynamic stereoscopy (Honegger, 1966), a very particular requirement, when it comes to pinpoint landing.

Visual senses and oculomotoricity would be overtaxed in all respects, when it comes to sonic or supersonic speed. High cruising speeds would not leave sufficient time for a full processing by visual senses. A flight distance (blind path) of 300 to 500 m was found to lie between retinal irritation and reaction in sonic speed travel, with accommodation, ocular movement, binocular fusion, and fixation being uncounted for.

Dynamic stereoacuity plays an important role in several sport disciplines

(Römhild, 1983; Trachtmann, 1973). There is an unambiguous need for prompt and accurate three-dimensional localisation in ball games, long and high jump, ski jumping, cross-country skiing, and gliding. Demands for accuracy are continuously arising in top competitive sports, and it would, therefore, be certainly useful to introduce dynamic stereoacuity testing for the selection of athletes in some sports. It should be done at sport centres, prior to specific practice of coaching programmes.

Good dynamic stereoacuity will also facilitate grasping, since the human hand movement must be visually controlled (Noll, 1973).

The view has been rapidly gaining ground that classical methods of ophthalmology are no longer sufficient for the adequate assessment of sophisticated performances of the visual process (Schober, 1972, 1976) and that examination methods would be needed by which several activities of the central nervous system could be tested and verified in combination (Backman, 1972). The need for testing of dynamic stereoacuity, i.e. dynamic stereoscopy and dynamic parallactoscopy, is, basically, supported by all the reasons given by examiners of monocular dynamic visual acuity and taken by them as the point of departure for their own investigations. The most important of these reasons relates to the existence of only loose correlations between static and dynamic visual activities (Weissmann and Freeburn, 1965).

Critical appraisal of the methods used for testing the visual sense in examinations relating to occupational and transport medicine has been correctly demanded by Schober (1972) as well as by Comberg (1953) and Otto and Höllmüller (1969), with the view to obtaining close-to-reality data. According to them, the sensorial system should be left as far as possible in its inseparable physiological interconnection with concomitant oculomotor activities. Hering pointed out, as early as 1879, that vision by the static eye would actually be an unnatural condition which we should require from our visual organ only for the purpose of medical examination. Dynamic vision testing would certainly enable a better assessment of vision (Methling and Wernicke, 1969; Söllner, 1961). There are very few occupational activities in which excellent three-dimensional vision only is necessary for the observation of static objects.

The great number of research papers on dynamic visual acuity is likely to support the assumption that dynamic stereoacuity will be included, in the not too remote future, in ophthalmological examination practice for certain trades and professions where high-quality three-dimensional vision of moving objects is essential, as well as for a more thorough elucidation of the failures that ought to be clearly stated in expert opinions. It has certainly not been accidental that earliest systematic investigations of dynamic visual acuity were not conducted for sensophysiological or clinical interests, but were undertaken by Ludvigh (1949) and Ludvigh and Miller (1958) for the practice-related requirements on naval aviator cadets.

The binocular rotational prismometer, as well as the parallactoscopometer, together with their triple-bar and quadruple-bar tests, can be easily designed and composed. Hence, there would be only a few obstacles to incorporating dynamic stereoacuity into fitness verification programmes for certain activities, particularly as tests of that kind would have to be made at only a few centres of occupational and sports medicine. The statement made by Honegger, Schäfer, and Jaeger (1969) with regard to visual acuity in the context of moving objects, would equally apply to the analysis of dynamic stereoacuity regarding both the sensophysiological fundamentals and the consequences for occupational medicine: 'Growing interest is being devoted at present to visual acuity for moving objects. There can be no doubt that such functional examination of visual acuity will greatly add to our knowledge on eye performance.'

This would be in keeping with the demand made as recently as 1984 by a newly established WHO Working Party (Regional Bureau for Europe) dealing with the problems of traffic accidents caused by medical factors, as well as with gaps in our knowledge in that context. This group of experts has emphasised that testing static perception only is insufficient and that dynamic vision with stereoscopic visual acuity is of major importance in the prevention of accidents.

No matter what future developments take place in this area, the results communicated in this paper should have clearly demonstrated that sensomotoricity is an important factor in detailed orientation on situations and on movements of objects in the third dimension. This sensomotricity is very sensitive to interference by disturbing factors. The impairment of dynamic stereoacuity cannot be effectively measured and elucidated by means of the routine methods so far used in ophthalmology.

Bibliography

1. Adamson J (1951): Ocular scanning and depth perception. Nature (London) 168: 345–347.
2. Aichmaier H (1983): Die Bedeutung des Stereosehens im Alltag. In: Schielbehandlung 14: 64–71.
3. Anderson EE, Weymouth FW (1923): I. Retinal mean local sign – an explanation of the fineness of binocular perception of distance. Am J Physiol 64: 561–567.
4. Andree G (1977): Die Leistungsfähigkeit des beidäugigen Sehns. Wehrmed Wschr 21: 304–308.
5. Anstis SM, Reinhardt-Rutland AH (1976): Interactions between motion aftereffects and induced movement. Vision Res 16: 1391–1394.
6. Aschenbrenner CM (1954): Problems in getting informations into and out of air photographs. Photogramm Engng 20: 398–401.
7. Aulhorn E (1971): Psychophysische Grundlagen des Binokularsehens. Bericht 4. Kongr Dtsch Ges Kbern. Berlin/Heidelberg/New York: Springer, pp 262–275.
8. Aulhorn E (1976): Funktionsprüfung des Auges zur Festsellung der Kraftfahreignung. In: Straub W (ed), Die ophthalmologischen Untersuchungsmethoden, Vol 2. Stuttgart: Enke, pp 922–990.
9. Aust W (1978): Fusionsbreitenbestimmung bei monokular und binokular reduziertem Visus Klin Mbl Augenheilk 173: 671–674.
10. Avetissov ES (1978): Diploptik – Ein prinzipiell neues System der Behandlung des Strabismus concomitans. Klin Mbl Augenheilk 172: 686–694.
11. Backman H (1972): Monocular and binocular visual ability in nocturnal driving visibility. Am J Optometry 49: 680–684.
12. Banks MS, Aslin RN, Letson RD (1975): Sensitive period for the development of human binocular vision. Science 190: 675–677.
13. Baumgartner F (1978): Sinnes- und neurophysiologische Organisationsprinzipien des visuellen Systems. Klin Mbl Augenheilk 173: 457–464.
14. Behrens F, Grüsser OJ (1977): Bewegungswahrnehmung und Augenbewegungen bei Flickerbelichtung unbewegter visueller Muster. Sitzungsbericht DOG. Neurophysiologie und Klinik der Augenbewegungsstörungen. Symposium Freiburg/ Breisgau.
15. Best F (1949): Zur Prüfung des stereoskopisch-räumlichen Sehens. Graefes Arch Ophthal 149: 413–430.
16. van Beuningen E (1949): Die Änderung von Sinnesleistungen durch Übung in ihrer Bedeutung für klinisch-ophthalmologische Untersuchungen. Graefes Arch Ophthal 149: 460–489.
17. Bishop PO (1975): Binocular vision. In: Adler's physiology of the eye. St. Louis: Mosby, 6th ed, pp 558–614.
18. Bishop PO (1977): Orientation and position disparities in stereopsis. In: Cool SJ, Smith EL (eds), Frontiers in visual science. New York/Heidelberg/Berlin: Springer, pp 176–189.
19. Blake R (1977): Spatial vision in the cat. In: Cool SJ, Smith EL (eds), Frontiers in visual science. New York/Heidelberg/Berlin: Springer, pp 209–217.

20. Bockelmann WD (1982): Auge, Brille, Auto. Basel: Karger.
21. Bourdy C (1974): L'acuité stéréoscopique, test de correspondance rétinienne normale, étude ses variations dans la région fovéale. Ann Oculist (Paris) 207: 651–661.
22. Broschmann D (1977): Sehstörungen und Kraftfahrtauglichkeit. Wiss Z Humboldt-Univ (Berlin) 26: 205–206.
23. Broschmann D (1981): Spezielle Probleme bei Sehanforderungen im Verkehrswesen. Auge und Beruf. Wiss Beitr Friedrich-Schiller-Univ (Jena): 155.
24. Broschmann D (1982): Methodenoptimierung bei der MDV-augenärztlichen Tauglichkeitsuntersuchung. Verkehrsmed 29: 95–100.
25. Burg A (1964): An investigation of some relationship between dynamic visual acuity, static visual and driving record. Report Univ California 64: 18.
26. Burg A (1965): Apparatus for measurement of dynamic visual acuity. Perc and Motor skills 20: 231–233.
27. Burg A (1966): Visual acuity as measured by dynamic and static tests. J Appl Psychol 50: 460–466.
28. Campos EC, Enoch JM (1980): Amount of aniseikonia compatible with fine binocular vision some old and new concepts. J pediat Ophthal 17: 44–47.
29. Chevaleraud JP, Brenneisen Ch, Santucci FG (1975): Etude comparative des résultats au Wirt, au stéréoscope et au TNO. Bull Soc Ophtal Fr 75: 757–760.
30. Colajanni G (1939): Visione binoculare e pereezione della profondità. Riv med. aeronaut 2: 240–246.
31. Colenbrander MC (1949): The accuracy of depth-perception the through movement parallax. Ophthalmologica (Basel) 118: 1039–1041.
32. Comberg W (1953): Blickfeld und Umblickfeld des Auges. Ber Dtsch Ophthal Ges 58: 6–15.
33. Cords R (1912): Bemerkungen zur Untersuchung des Tiefenschätzungsvermögens. Z Augenheilk 27: 346–354.
34. Creuzfeldt O (1979): Repräsentation der visuellen Umwelt im Gehirn. Verh Dtsche Zool Ges (Stuttgart) 1979: 5–18.
35. Crone RA (1973): Diplopia. Amsterdam: Excerpta Medica.
36. Davidson M (1935): A simple device for measuring stereopsis. Am J Ophthal 18: 356.
37. de Decker W, Haase W (1976): Subnormales Binokularsehen – Versuch einer Einteilung des Mikrostrabismus. Klin Mbl Augenheilk 169: 182–195.
38. de Decker W, Scheffel T (1978): Simultaneous investigation of fixation disparity, stereothreshold and horopter balance. Graefes Arch Ophthal 207: 97–109.
39. Dehler H (1967): Sehschärfe und verwandte Fragen. In: 10 Jahre Forschung für besseres Sehen. Institut für med Optik (München) 1967: 78–86.
40. Dieker P, Honegger H (1968): Registrierungen von kreisförmigen Augenbewegungen. Ber Dtsch Ophthal Ges 68: 477–479.
41. Ditchburn RW, Ginsborg BL (1953): Involuntary eye movement during fixation. J Psychol 119: 1–19.
42. Doege E, Krause O (1977): Ein neuer Weg zur binokularen Funktionsprüfung. Folia Ophthal 2: 199–202.
43. Dowrick PW (1975): Stereopsis maintained with identical stimulation to both eyes. Quart J exp Psychol 27: 479–486.
44. Drischel H (1961): Über den fixationsregelnden Apparat des menschlichen Auges. In: Mittelstaedt H (ed), Regelvorgänge in lebenden Wesen. München: Oldenbourg.
45. Dubois-Poulsen A (1968): La fatigue visuelle. 3rd Eur Congres Hist Ophthalmol (Amsterdam) 157–161.
46. Ebbecke U (1948): Über eine Umwandlung des Gesichtsfeldes bei Dauerexposition. Pflügers Arch Physiol 249: 87–93.
47. Feldes D, Römhild H (1981): Kritik an der Durchführung des 3-Stäbchentests. Folia Ophthal 6: 55–59.

48. Florentini A, Maffei L (1970): Electrophysiological evidence for binocular disparity detectors in human visual system. Science 169: 208–211.
49. Forbös TW, Snyder TE, Pain RF (1965): Traffic sign requirements. Review of factors involved, previous studies and needed research. Highway Research Record 70: 48–54.
50. Forde J, MacKinnon GE (1975): Binocular stimulation and the fragmentation of after-images. Quart J exp Psychol 27: 565–577.
51. Fox R (1977): Binocularity and stereopsis in the evolution of vertebrate vision. In: Cool SJ, Smith EL (eds), Frontiers in visual science. New York/Heidelberg/Berlin: pp 316–325.
52. Frejman SI (1940): Physiologische Normen er Sehschärfe des Tiefensehens in die Ferne mit Hilfe des Tiefensehmessers [in Russian]. Vestn Oftalm 16: 262–269.
53. Frey RG (1977): Auge und Verkehr. Bücherei des Augenarztes Vol 71. Stuttgart: Enke.
54. Frey RG (1953): Die Beziehung zur Sehschärfe und Tiefensehschärfe. Wien med Wschr 1953: 436–438.
55. Friedburg D (1980): Abnehmende lokale Stereopsis mit zunehmender Querdisparation, ein Hinweis auf abnehmende Dichte der binokularen Projektion am Rande des Panumareals. Graefes Arch Ophthal 213: 109–114.
56. Frisby JP, Mein J, Saye A, Stanworth A (1975): Use of random dot stereograms in the clinical assessment of strabismic patients. Br J Ophthal 59: 545–552.
57. Fruböese A, Jaensch PA (1923): Der Einfluß verschiedener Faktoren auf die Tiefensehschärfe. Z Biol 78: 119–131.
58. Gehrke G (1965): Tagungsber 5. Militärmedizin Kongreß Verkehrsmed 12: 322–324.
59. Geratewohl SJ (1954): Die Physiologie des Menschen im Flugzeug. München: Barth.
60. Giardini A (1949): Einfluß des Alkohols auf die Tätigkeit der Fusion von Netzhautbildern [in Italian]. Giorn ital oftalm 2: 446–451.
61. Gibson JJ (1966): The senses considered as perceptual systems. New York: Houghton, Mifflin & Co.
62. Glees M (1949): Über den Einfluß der Tiefenwahrnehmung auf das Sehen im Dunkeln. Graefes Arch Ophthal 149: 680–685.
63. Gramberg-Danielsen B (1976): Verkehrsophthalmologie. In: Velhagen K (ed), Der Augenarzt, Vol 4. Leipzig: Thieme, 2nd ed, pp 287–478.
64. Grosslight JH, Fletcher JJ, Masterton RB, Hagen R (1978): Monocular vision and landing performance in general aviation pilots: cyclops revisited. Hum Factors 20: 27–32.
65. Haase HJ (1980): Binokulare Korrektion. Düsseldorf: Schrickel.
66. Haberkorn R (1965): Die Verbesserung der Tiefensehschärfe durch monokular vorgesetzte Lichtabsorptions- und Farbfilter. Med Fak Leipzig, Dissertation.
67. Harter MR, Towle VL, Zakrzewski M, Moyer SM (1977): An objective indicant of binocular vision in humans size-specific interocular suppression of visual evoked potentials. Electroenceph clin Neurophysiol 43: 825–836.
68. Hartmann E, Stöcker L (1983): Die Bedeutung des querdisparaten Tiefensehens am Arbeitsplatz und im Straßenverkehr. Fortschr Ophthalm 80: 496–497.
69. Hass HD (1982): Kopfschmerz und Auge. In: Sachsenweger R (ed), Neuroophthalmologie. Leipzig: Thieme, 3rd ed, pp 507–513.
70. Heine L (1900): Sehschärfe und Tiefenwahrnehmung. Graefes Arch Ophthal 51: 146–158.
71. Heinsius E (1947): Über die sekundären Faktoren des binokularen räumlichen Tiefensehens. Graefes Arch Ophthal 147: 1–16.
72. Heinsius E (1958): Über Raumwahrnehmung und Eisenbahndienst. Ärztl Dienst DB 10: 274–277.
73. Heinsius E (1964): Sehorgan und Verkehrssicherheit. Ärztl Dienst DB 25: 53–61.
74. Hell W (1978): Movement parallax: an asymptotic function of amplitude and velocity of head motion. Vision Res 18: 629–635.
75. Helmer R (1972): Experimentelle Untersuchungen zur Fahrtüchtigkeit nach Einnahme von Haschisch. Blutalkohol 9: 213.

76. von Helmholtz H (1910): Handbuch der Physiologischen Optik, Vol 3: Die Lehre von den Gesichtswahrnehmungen. Hamburg/Leipzig: Voss, 3rd ed.
77. Helveston EM, von Noorden GK (1967): Microtropia. Arch Ophthal (Chicago) 78: 272–277.
78. Hering E (1879): Der Raumsinn und die Bewegungen des Auges. In: Hermann L (ed), Handbuch der Physiologie, Vol III/1. Leipzig.
79. Herzau V (1976): Stereosehen bei alternierender Bildarbietung. Graefes Arch Ophthal 200: 85–91.
80. Heydenreich A, Wittwer B (1981): Berufs- und Fahrtauglichkeit von einäugig gewordenen Patienten. Auge und Beruf. Wiss Beitr Friedrich-Schiller-Univ (Jena) pp 172–174.
81. Hofmann FB (1925): Die Lehre vom Raumsinn des Auges. In: Graefe-Saemisch, Handbuch der gesamten Augenheilkunde, III: Physiologische Optik, Teil 2, Berlin/Heidelberg/New York: Springer, 2nd ed.
82. Hofstetter HW, Bertsch JD (1976): Does stereoscopic change with age? Am J Optom physiol Optics 53: 664–667.
83. Holland G (1960): Binokularsehen und anomale Netzhautkorrespondenz bei kleinem Schielwinkel. Klin Mbl Augenheilk 137: 786–797.
84. Höllhubert J, Aigner JC, Kastenhuber M (1975): Die Selbsteinschätzung von Alter, Aufmerksamkeitsumfang und Rigiditätsfaktoren. Z Verkehrsrecht 20: 92–96.
85. Honegger H (1966): Einige ophthalmologische Aspekte der Flugmedizin. Der med Sachverständige 62: 262–274.
86. Honegger H (1970): Untersuchungen von Koordinationsstörungen des Auges mit Hilfe der Sehschärfe für bewegte Objekte. Ber Dtsch Ophthal Ges 70: 294–299.
87. Honegger H, Alexandridis E (1970): Sehschärfe für bewegte Objekte in Abhängigkeit von der Adaptation. Graefes Arch Ophthal 181: 1–11.
88. Honegger H, Kampschulte R, Klein H (1970): Störung der Sehschärfe für bewegte Objekte durch Alkohol. Blutalkohol 7: 31–44.
89. Honegger H, Schäfer WD (1964): Registrierung von Augenbewegungen als Beitrag zur Untersuchung der Sehschärfe für bewegte Objekte. Graefes Arch Ophthal 166: 601–616.
90. Honegger H, Schäfer WD (1968): Sehschärfe für bewegte Objekte. Einige Gesichtspunkte für die Verkehrsmedizin. Zbl Verkehrs-Med 14: 160–167.
91. Honegger H, Schäfer WD (1968): Sehschärfe für bewegte Objekte bei Blickhebung und Blicksenkung. Ber Dtsch Ophthal Ges 68: 419–426.
92. Honegger H, Schäfer WD (1970): Funktionelle Untersuchung des Blickfeldes mit Hilfe der Sehschärfe für bewegte Objekte. Klin Mbl Augenheilk 157: 801–806.
93. Honegger H, Schäfer WD, Jaeger W (1969): Vergleich von horizontaler und kreisförmiger Projektion der Sehzeichen. Graefes Arch Ophthal 178: 132–146.
94. Hoogerheide J (1964): Preliminary report concerning peripheral dynamic vision. Aeromed Acta (Soesterberg) 9: 139–142.
95. Howard HJ (1919): A test for judgement of distance. Trans Am Ophthal Soc 17: 195–235.
96. Hubel DH, Wiesel TN (1962): Receptive fields, binocular interaction and functional architecture in the cat's visual cortex. J Physiol 160: 106–154.
97. Hübler B (1964): Untersuchungen über die Sehschärfe für bewegte Objekte bei horizontaler Projektion der Sehzeichen. Med Fak Heidelberg, Dissertation.
98. Jaeger W (1958): Sehschärfe für bewegte Objekte. Klin Mbl Augenheilk 133: 436.
99. Jaeger W, Honegger H (1964): Der Einfluß von Augenkrankheiten auf die Sehschärfe für bewegte Objekte. Graefes Arch Ophthal 166: 583–600.
100. Jeansch ER (1911): Über die Wahrnehmung des Raumes. Z Physiol, Suppl Vol 6.
101. Jaensch ER (1939): Neues and Grundsätzliches zu den Aufgaben der Wahrnehmungspsychologie. Z Psychol 146: 193–228.
102. Jameson D, Hurvich LM (1959): Note on factors influencing the relation between stereoscopic acuity and observation distance. J Opt Soc Am 49: 639–642.
103. Jofe Z (1937): Tiefensehen bei Anisometropen. Vestn Oftal 10: 423–425.

104. Julesz B (1964): Binocular depth perception without familiarity cues. Science 145: 356–362.
105. Keidel WD (1976): Allgemeine Sinnesphysiologie, visuelles System. Berlin/Heidelberg/New York: Springer, 2nd ed.
106. Kessler J (1947): Vorrichtung zur Messung der Tiefensehschärfe. Klin Mbl Augenheilk 112: 339–341.
107. Kienle G (1968): Die optischen Wahrnehmungsstörungen und die nichteuklidische Struktur des Sehraumes. Stuttgart: Thieme.
108. Kirijakoff K, Wassilewa M, Raitschewa W (1964): Über einige Komplex-Methoden zur dynamischen Untersuchung der Ermüdung bei Dispatchern und Lokführern. Zbl Verkehrsmed 11: 343–348.
109. Kitte G, Dieroff HG (1971): Zur Problematik der Farbsinnänderung unter Lärmimission. Klin Mbl Augenheilk 158: 732–739.
110. Körner F, Dichgans J (1968): Bewegungswahrnehmung, optokinetischer Nystagmus and retinale Bildwanderung. Graefes Arch Ophthal 174: 34–48.
111. Krause E, Hempel W (1982): Untersuchungen zum Binokularsehen bei psychische Kranken. Folia Ophthal 7: 191–194.
112. Kroj G (1972): Der Einfluß des Alters auf Risikobereitschaft und Sicherheitseinstellung – eine Fragebogenerhebung. Z Verkehrssicherheit 18: 107–109.
113. Kronesser H (1981): Blendung im Straßenverkehr unter dynamischen Bedingungen. Augenoptik 98: 105–107.
114. Krot LP (1972): Determination of visual acuity with movable lines in the disc of Roth's apparatus [in Russian]. Oftal Z 27: 310–311.
115. Krudewig M (1953): Die Lehren von der visuellen Wahrnehmung und Vorstellung bei ER Jaensch und seinen Schülern. Glan: Meisenheim.
116. Kühner G (1958): Untersuchungen über die Sehschärfe für bewegte Objekte. Med Fak Heidelberg, Dissertation.
117. Lang J (1982): Mikrostrabismus. Stuttgart: Enke, 2nd ed.
118. Lang J (1983): Ein neuer Stereotest. Fortschr Ophthalmol 80: 269–270.
119. Langlands NMS (1929): Experiments on binocular vision. Report upon the physiology of vision. Brighton: Wright and Sons.
120. Langmuir J (1938): Motion and visual acuity. Science 105: 176–178.
121. van Lear P, Blum K, Niesel P (1978): Zur Brauchbarkeit des 'Random Dot Tests' für schulärztliche Untersuchungen. Klin Mbl Augenheilk 172: 635–638.
122. Lehmann D, Julesz B (1978): Lateralized cortical potentials evoked in humans by dynamic random-dot stereograms. Vision Res 18: 1265.
123. Lehmkuhle SW, Fox R (1975): Effect of binocular rivalry suppression on the motion aftereffect. Vision Res 15: 855–859.
124. Leopoldsberger W (1942): Über die Beeinflußbarkeit des Fusionsvermögens durch äußere Faktoren. Wien Klin Wschr pp 705–706.
125. Letourneau JE, Millodot M (1974): The effect of noise on visual fields. Eye, Ear, Nose, Throat Monthly 53: 49–51.
126. Levy NS, Glick EB (1974): Stereoscopic perception and Snellen visual acuity. Am J Ophthal 78: 722–724.
127. Levy MM, Lawson RB (1978): Stereopsis and binocular rivalry from dichoptic stereograms. Vision Res 18: 239–246.
128. Lieschke HJ (1982): Intoxikationen. In: Sachsenweger R (ed), Neuroophthalmologie. Leipzig: Thieme, 3rd ed.
129. Litinski GA (1936): Normen der Schärfe des Tiefensehens bei Normalsichtigen (Erwachsenen) am Stereomyograph (in Russian). Vestn Oftal 9: 661–673.
130. Lorenz R (1943): Binokulares Raumsehen und Refraktion. Klin Mbl Augenheilk 109: 660–669.
131. Low F (1947): The peripheral motion acuity of 50 subjects. Am J Physiol 148: 124–131.

132. Ludvigh E (1949): Visual acuity while one is viewing a moving object. Arch Ophthal (Chicago) 42: 14–22.
133. Ludvigh E, Miller JW (1958): Study of visual acuity during the ocular pursuit of moving test objects. J Opt Soc Am 48: 799–802.
134. Lücking GH, Struppler A (1982): Neurologische Alterungsprozesse und ihr Einfluß auf das Verhalten älterer Menschen am Steuer. Neues Optikerjournal 24(6): 23–25.
135. Lyle TK, Bridgeman GJO (1959): Worth and Chavasse's squint. London, 9th ed.
136. Mackay DM (1970): Perception and brain function. In: Schmitt FO et al (eds), The neurosciences II study program. New York: Rockefeller University Press, pp 303–316.
137. Manz R (1939/40): Der Einfluß geringer Alkoholgaben auf Teilfunktionen von Auge und Ohr. Dtsch Z ges gerichtl Med 32: 301–312.
138. Matsubayashi A (1937): Der Einfluß der Ortsveränderung der beobachteten Objekte bei der 2-Stäbchenmethode auf die Feinheit der Tiefenwahrnehmung und die physiologische Nullstellung. Acta Soc Ophthal Jap. 41: 2257–2268.
139. Mayer HB, Lane JC (1973): Monocular pilots: a follow-up-study. Aerospace Med 44: 1070–1074.
140. Mayer MJ (1977): Development of anisotropy in late childhood. Vision Res 17: 703–710.
141. Mehlhose F (1975): Modifizierter 3-Stäbchen-Test auf elektromechanischer Grundlage. Augenspiegel 21: 276–278.
142. Merté HJ (1978): Die Bedeutung der Ergophthalmologie. Arbeitsmed Sozialmed Präv-Med 13: 89–93.
143. Merté HJ (1985): citation. in: Neues Optikerjournal 1985(6): 38.
144. Methling D, Wernicke J (1969): Die Eigenschaften des Auges beim Sehen bewegter Objekte. Augenoptik 96: 13–19.
145. Micko HC (1955/56): Untersuchungen der Tiefensehschärfe für größere Entfernungen. Z Psychol 3: 530–538.
146. Miller JW (1958): Study of visual acuity during the ocular pursuit of moving test objects. J Opt Soc Am 48: 803.
147. Miller JW, Ludvigh E (1962): The effect of relative motion on visual acuity. Surv Ophthal 7: 83–116.
148. Miwa T, Terada K, Morita S, Yamada T, Suzumura A (1972): Human perception-response to a moving object in terms of pursuit movement of the eye. Ann Rep Environm Med Nagoya Univ 19: 35–40.
149. Monjé M (1947): Über die Beziehungen des Stereoeffektes zur Tiefensehschärfe. Pflügers Arch 249: 377–384.
150. Monjé M (1949): Zur Prüfung des stereoskopisch-räumlichen Sehens. Graefes Arch Ophthal 149: 413–430.
151. Monjé M (1969): Lichtsinn, Physiologie des Auges. In: Velhagen K (ed), Der Augenarzt Vol 1. Leipzig: Thieme, 2nd ed., pp 173–288.
152. Münster C (1942): Über einige Probleme der stereoskopischen Messung. Z Instrumentenkunde 62: 346–357.
153. Noda H (1975): Depression in the excitability of relay cells of lateral geniculate nucleus following saccadic eye movements in the cat. J Physiol 249: 87–102.
154. Noll G (1973): Zur Bedeutung des räumlichen Sehens und des Schielens für den Betriebsdienst. Ärztl Dienst 34: 168–169.
155. von Noorden GK (1979): Zur Entstehung der Amblyopie, experimentelle Untersuchungen. Ber Dtsch Ophthal Ges 77: 815–817.
156. Ogle KN (1958): Note on stereoscopic acuity and observation distance. J Opt Soc Am 48: 794–798.
157. Oloff W, Podesta H (1937): Die Funktionsprüfung des Auges unter besonderer Berücksichtigung der Störungen des Farbensinnes. Berlin: Springer, 2nd ed.
158. Otto J, Höllmüller O (1969): Klinische Untersuchungen zur Labilität der Binokularfunktionen. Klin Mbl Augenheilk 155: 721–743.

159. Over R, Broerse J, Crassini B, Lovegrove W (1973): Spatial determinants of the aftereffect of seen motion. Vision Res 13: 1681–1690.
160. Perlia R (1911): Ein vereinfachtes Stereoskopometer. Klin Mbl Augenheilk 49(2): 492–494.
161. Pettigrew JD (1979): Binocular visual processing in the owl's telencephalon. Proc Roy Soc Lond B 204: 435–454.
162. Pfalz G (1907): Ein verbesserter Stereoskoptometer zur Prüfung des Tiefenschätzungsvermögens. Klin Mbl Augenheilk 45(2): 85–95.
163. Pierce DM, Benton, AL (1975): Relationship between monocular and binocular depth acuity. Ophthalmologica (Basel) 170: 43–50.
164. Piper HF (1951): Der Einfluß des Adaptationszustandes auf Ablauf unwillkürlicher Augenbewegungen. Ber Dtsch Ophthal Ges 57: 260–265.
165. Piper HF (1969): Optische Orientierung im Straßenverkehr und ihre Untersuchungsmethoden. Med Klinik 64: 1092–1098.
166. Pulfrich E (1922): Die zu einer Gesichtswahrnehmung nötige Zeit und die Art des Anstiegs der Lichtempfindung. Naturw 10: 571–573.
167. Regan D, Beverley KI (1978): Illusory motion in depth: aftereffect of adaptation to changing size. Vision Res 18: 209–212.
168. Regan D, Beverley KI, Cynader M (1979): Stereoscopic subsystems for position in depth and for motion in depth. Proc Roy Soc Lond B 204: 485–501.
169. Regan D, Spekreijse H (1970): Electrophysiological correlate of binocular depth perception in man. Nature (London) 225: 92–94.
170. Reinecke RD, Simons K (1974): A new stereoscopic test for amblyopia screening. Am J Ophthal 78: 714–721.
171. Rennert H (1977): Störungen der tiefenräumlichen Wahrnehmung und Wiedergabe. Nova Acta Leopoldina (Halle), No. 228, Vol. 47.
172. Roggenkämper P (1983): Stereosehen bei vermindertem Visus. Klin Mbl Augenheilk 183: 105–109.
173. Römhild H (1978): Beurteilung der Sportfähigkeit und körperlichen Belastung bei Störungen des beidäugigen Sehens. Medizin and Sport 18: 337–340.
174. Römhild H (1983): Beiträge zum stereoskopischen Sehen für Theorie und Praxis. Magdeburg, Promotion-B-Arbeit (med.).
175. Rüssel A (1939): Die Übbarkeit des binokularen Tiefensehens. Ber Dtsch Ges Psychol pp 254–257.
176. Sachsenweger M (1983): Erste Untersuchungsergebnisse über die Stereo-Sehschärfe für bewegte Objekte. Klin Mbl Augenheilk 182: 65–67.
177. Sachsenweger M (1984/85): Das Phänomen der unterschiedlichen Tiefensehschärfe beim Sehen in Nähe und Ferne. In: Tost M (ed), Aktuelle Probleme der Strabologie. Halle – Wittenberg: Martin-Luther-Univ Wiss. Beiträge, pp 99–102.
178. Sachsenweger R (1954): Die Tiefensehschärfe bei herabgesetzter Beleuchtung. Graefes Arch Ophthal 155: 496.
179. Sachsenweger R (1955): Experimentelle Untersuchungen über den Einfluß der Ermüdung auf das räumliche Sehen. Dtsch Z gerichtl Med 44: 66–76.
180. Sachsenweger R (1958): Experimentelle und klinische Untersuchungen des stereoskopischen Raumes. Leipzig.
181. Sachsenweger R (1972): Pathologie und Klinik der Refraktionsanomalien. In: Velhagen K (ed), Der Augenarzt, Vol 2. Leipzig: Thieme, pp 713–1006.
182. Samsonova VG (1936): Einfluß der Objektform auf das stereoskopische Sehen. Graefes Arch Ophthal 135: 30–48.
183. Sanders Th (1970): Der Führerschein auf Zeit – Juristische Gesichtspunkte. Z Verkehrssicherheit 16: 170–186.
184. Schaefer H, Ebner F (1948): Über einen neuen Stereoeffekt und die Tiefensehschärfe. Pflügers Arch 249: 637–654.

185. Schmidt T (1976): Zur Prüfung der Sehfunktion in der Dämmerung zwecks Feststellung der Fahrtauglichkeit im Straßenverkehr. Ophthalmologica (Basel) 172: 160–165.
186. Schneider G (1981): Sehschärfe und Binokularfunktion bei beidseitiger Pseudophakie. Klin Mbl Augenheilk 178: 149.
187. Schober H (1954): Das Sehen, Vol 2. Leipzig: Fachbuchverlag.
188. Schober H (1972): Methodenkritik der Fahrtauglichkeitsuntersuchungen am Beispiel der Überprüfung des Gesichtssinnes. Med Welt NF 23: 426–429.
189. Schober H (1976): Prüfung der Sehfunktionen. In: Straub W (ed), Die ophthalmologischen Untersuchungsmethoden, Vol 2. Stuttgart: Enke, pp 273–327.
190. Schober H, Munker H, Grimm W (1967): Zur Erkennbarkeit bewegter Objekte: Dynamische Sehschärfe. Klin Mbl Augenheilk 151: 399–402.
191. Schott G, Seidel K (1982): Psychopharmakotherapie. Berlin: Volk and Gesundheit.
192. Schüler H, Mürmel G (1979): Untersuchungen über die durch die Frontkarosserie von Personenkraftwagen verursachten Gesichtsfeldausfälle. Verkehrsmed 26: 225–229.
193. Schulz E, Schulz G (1974): Die Raumwahrnehmungsstörungen bei psychiatrischen Erkrankungen. Halle, Dissertation.
194. Schumann Ch (1959): Das stereoskopische Sehen im Verkehr. Bahnarzt 6: 292–299.
195. Scott WE, Mash J (1974): Stereoacuity in normal individuals. Ann Ophthal 6: 99–101.
196. von Seelen W (1983): Was geschieht im Gehirn mit den Bildern beider Augen? Aschaffenburger Kontaktlinsentagung 16: 5–12.
197. Shipley T (1971): The first random-dot stereogram. Vision Res 11: 1491–1492.
198. Siebeck R (1955): Akkommodationsasymmetrien. Ber Dtsch Ophthal Ges 59: 247–251.
199. Söllner G (1961): Zur Formenempfindlichkeit des Auges bei Beobachtung bewegter Objekte. Karlsruhe, Dissertation.
200. Srinivasan MV, Bernard GD (1975): The effect of motion on visual acuity of the compound eye: a theoretical analysis. Vision Res 15: 545–525.
201. Strelow ER, Day RH (1975): Visual movement aftereffect: evidence for independent adaptation to moving target and stationary surround. Vision Res 15: 117–121.
202. Suzumura A (1964): Studies on the visual acuity: the kinetic visual acuity for the visual objects of colored light. Ann Rep Environ Med Nagoya Univ 12: 53–60.
203. Syka J (1979): Neurophysiologische Grundlagen des Bewegungsschens. In: Drischel H, Kirmse W (eds), Das okulomotorische System. Leipzig, pp 13–20.
204. Teichner WH, Kobrick JL, Wehrkamp RF (1955): The effects of terrain and observation distance on relative depth discrimination. Am J Psychol 68: 193–208.
205. Teping C, Pesch T (1984): Untersuchungen zum Nachweis der Stereopsis durch Ableitung visuell evozierter kortikaler Potentiale (VECP). Fortschr Ophthalmol 81: 480–482.
206. Toppel W (1976): Heterophorie und Antidepressiva. Klin Mbl Augenheilk 169: 138.
207. Tost M, Krüger KE (1979): Physiologische und methodische Grundlagen der Pleoptik und Orthoptik. Leipzig: Thieme, 3rd ed.
208. Trachtman JN (1973): The relationship between ocular motilities and batting average in little leaguers. Am J Optometry 50: 914–919.
209. von Tschermak A (1931): Optischer Raumsinn. Handbuch der normalen und pathologischen Physiologie 12/2, 912ff, 940–950.
210. von Tschermak A (1939): Über Parallaktoskopie. Pflügers Arch Physiol 241: 455–469.
211. von Tschermak A (1947): Einführung in die physiologische Optik. Vienna: Springer, 2nd ed.
212. Tyler CW, Sutter EE (1979): Depth from spatial frequency difference: an old kind of stereopsis? Vision Res 19: 859–865.
213. Ueberschaar G (1975): Das binokulare Sehen. Augenoptik 91: 53–57.
214. Ueberschaar G (1976): Optologie, Grundzüge der Lehre vom Sehen. Rathenow: Duncker.
215. Verhoeff FH (1933): An improved and a new test for stereoscopic vision. Am J Ophthal 16: 589–591.

216. Vesper G (1965): Über die Qualität der Tiefensehschärfe beim Sehen in die Ferne unter den Bedingungen des Fahrdienstes der Eisenbahn. Verkehrsmed 12: 515–524.
217. Vokes E (1980): Auge und Alter – Untersuchungen von Heterophorie, Stereopsis und Zyklofusion an 70 Probanden aller Altersstufen. Bonn, Dissertation.
218. Vomberg HE, Skrandies W (1985): Untersuchungen des Stereoschens im Zufallspunktmuster-VECP: Normbefunde und klinische Anwendung. Klin Mbl Augenheilk 187: 205–208.
219. Wagner E (1949): Die Zeitschwelle der Tiefensehschärfe. Klin Mbl Augenheilk 114: 557–562.
220. Wäldrich B (1978): Untersuchungen des räumlichen Sehens psychisch Kranker mit einer polarisationsstereometrischen Methode. Halle, Med Dissertation.
221. Walther H, Uchtländer M, Meyer FP (1983): Zur Problematik 'Dosierung – Blutspiegel – Wirkung' in der Psychopharmakologie. Medicamentum 10/11: 285–288.
222. Weissmann S, Freeburne CM (1965): Visual acuity with moving test objects. J Exper Psychol 70: 141–146.
223. Westheimer G (1979): The spatial sense of the eye. Proctor lecture. Invest Ophthal Vis Sci 18: 893–897.
224. Westheimer G, McKee SP (1979): What prior uniocular processing is necessary for stereopsis? Invest Ophthal Vis Sci 18: 614–621.
225. Woodburne LS (1934): The effect of a constant visual angle upon the binocular discrimination of depth differences. Am J Psychol 46: 273–286.

Subject index

Monographs in Ophthalmology

1. P.C. Maudgal and L. Missotten (eds.): *Superficial Keratitis.* 1981
   ISBN 90-6193-801-5
2. P.F.J. Hoyng: *Pharmacological Denervation and Glaucoma.* A Clinical Trial Report with Guanethidine and Adrenaline in One Eyedrop. 1981
   ISBN 90-6193-802-3
3. N.W.H.M. Dekkers: *The Cornea in Measles.* 1981 ISBN 90-6193-803-1
4. P. Leonard and J. Rommel: *Lens Implantation.* 30 Years of Progress. 1982
   ISBN 90-6193-804-X
5. C.E. van Nouhuys: *Dominant Exudative Vitreoretinopathy and Other Vascular Developmental Disorders of the Peripheral Retina.* 1982 ISBN 90-6193-805-8
6. L. Evens (ed.): *Convergent Strabismus.* 1982 ISBN 90-6193-806-6
7. A. Neetens, A. Lowenthal and J.J. Martin (eds.): *The Visual System in Myelin Disorders.* 1984 ISBN 90-6193-807-4
8. H.J.M. Völker-Dieben: *The Effect of Immunological and Non-Immunological Factors on Corneal Graft Survival.* A Single Centre Study. 1984
   ISBN 90-6193-808-2
9. J.A. Oosterhuis (ed.): *Ophthalmic Tumours.* 1985 ISBN 90-6193-528-8
10. O. van Nieuwenhuizen: *Cerebral Visual Disturbance in Infantile Encephalopathy.* 1987 ISBN 0-89838-860-0
11. E.A.C.M. Sanders, R.J.W. de Keizer and D.S. Zee (eds.): *Eye Movement Disorders.* 1987 ISBN 0-89838-874-0
12. R. Živojnović: *Silicone Oil in Vitreoretinal Surgery.* 1987
    ISBN 0-89838-879-1
13. A. Brini, P. Dhermy and J. Sahel: *Oncology of the Eye and Adnexa.* Atlas of Clinical Pathology / *Oncologie de l'Œil et des Annexes.* Atlas Anatomo-Clinique / *Onkologische Diagnostik in der Ophthalmologie.* Vergleichender Klinisch-Pathologischer Atlas. 1990 ISBN 0-7923-0409-8
14. J.J. De Laey and M. Hanssens: *Vascular Tumors and Malformations of the Ocular Fundus.* 1990 ISBN 0-7923-0750-X

KLUWER ACADEMIC PUBLISHERS – DORDRECHT / BOSTON / LONDON

GPSR Compliance

The European Union's (EU) General Product Safety Regulation (GPSR) is a set of rules that requires consumer products to be safe and our obligations to ensure this.

If you have any concerns about our products, you can contact us on ProductSafety@springernature.com

In case Publisher is established outside the EU, the EU authorized representative is:

Springer Nature Customer Service Center GmbH
Europaplatz 3
69115 Heidelberg, Germany

Batch number: 10620141

Printed by Printforce, the Netherlands